Producing Patient-Centered
Health Care

Producing Patient-Centered Health Care

Patient Perspectives about Health and Illness and the Physician/Patient Relationship

James Monroe Smith

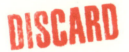

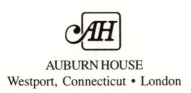

AUBURN HOUSE
Westport, Connecticut • London

Library of Congress Cataloging-in-Publication Data

Smith, James Monroe.
    Producing patient-centered health care : patient perspectives
about health and illness and the physician/patient relationship /
James Monroe Smith.
        p. cm.
    Includes bibliographical references and index.
    ISBN 0–86569–293–9 (alk. paper)
    1. Physician and patient.   2. Medicine and psychology.
3. Holistic medicine.   I. Title.
R727.3.S58   1999
610.69′6—dc21   99–12474

British Library Cataloguing in Publication Data is available.

Library of Congress Catalog Card Number: 99–12474
ISBN: 0–86569–293–9

First published in 1999

Auburn House, 88 Post Road West, Westport, CT 06881
An imprint of Greenwood Publishing Group, Inc.
www.greenwood.com

Printed in the United States of America

The paper used in this book complies with the
Permanent Paper Standard issued by the National
Information Standards Organization (Z39.48–1984).

10 9 8 7 6 5 4 3 2 1

This book is dedicated

- To all health care and medical professionals who put their patients' needs first and who passionately advocate for their patients' welfare—either in hospitals or the legislatures;

- To lay persons who advocate for and listen to other patients; and

- To caregivers the world over who provide the care required for loved ones.

And particularly to:

- Richard Garibaldi, M.D., my personal physician, who incorporates a holistic approach to health in his practice of medicine; and

- Jan McDonald, my cousin, who counsels many alcoholics and their families and who is always ready to assist those in need.

Contents

Preface

SOME PERSONAL THOUGHTS

I have observed the limitations of and the problems posed by the health care and medical establishments in my professional and personal life. I am a lawyer and was the founding executive director of the AIDS Legal Council of Chicago and, in that capacity, became aware of the personalities, hopes, dreams, fears, and coping mechanisms of persons facing a chronic/terminal illness.[1] My perspectives are also shaped by the fact that I have had acquired immunodeficiency syndrome (AIDS) since February 1995. The content and organization of this book, therefore, not only reflect my reading and my talks with patients and doctors, but also my personal experience of being admitted to the hospital, seeing my own physician, making outpatient visits (often monthly), thinking about my own death (and, as a result, executing my own will and advance directives, planning my own healing service, and writing my own obituary), dating men with human immunodeficiency virus/AIDS (HIV/AIDS), talking to debt collectors who almost universally have what I would consider incredibly rude tactics, and negotiating the sometimes dehumanizing public aid bureaucracy.[2]

Over the past few years, I have been a caregiver for aging parents—my mother has had Parkinsons's disease for 15 years and over the past year my father was diagnosed with and treated for bladder cancer. Since the three of us are all on Medicare (and my mother and I are on Medicaid) we have also received the services of the home health care "industry"—in our home, this has meant services (e.g., assistance with laundry, cooking, shopping, and "personal care" for my mother and father) provided by two different agencies and some 20 new individuals. Prior to that assistance with cooking and shopping, members of my church cooked meals and did some shopping and took my father to medical appointments with his urologist—a round trip of three hours from our home in rural Connecticut. My father's treatment with chemotherapy left him quite weak and "washed out" and for several months severely depressed, presumably as a result of his limitations and inability to work. I do not describe the sickness in our family to elicit any sympathy or to complain, but merely to illustrate that my experiences with people with illness and the systems that treat them are not superficial.

My own health was put in jeopardy by my caregiving duties and, at one point, I became aware that I was physically exhausted and had lost 10 pounds (with my normal weight about 125 pounds, this represented an 8 percent loss of body weight). To preserve my energy I limited my cooking, shopping, and taking my dad to the local doctor. At one point, I cancelled my mother's appointment with her neurologist because I did not have the energy to push her around in a wheelchair at the medical center—where my doctor is also located. In canceling the appointment I explained our family predicament. Consequently, it is critical for health care professionals (HCPs) to realize a family's situation even though a particular physician may be treating one member of that family.

My sister and a social worker from one of the home care agencies have been my parents' prime advocates for the timely receipt of services. I would not have had the sheer willpower or energy to do it alone. For example, I know it took my sister several weeks of advocacy to get one of the agencies to add about four hours per week so that aides could do additional shopping and cooking. And this advocacy was needed, even though my mother is a client of our state's "elder care program," in which she is assigned a case manager to coordinate (and advocate for) her care.

I believe the limitations of the health care and medical establishments are chiefly due to the failure of these systems to focus on the needs of patients and their caregivers. Rather, these establishments often focus on the convenience to HCPs. For example, HCPs often fail to inform those family members who are patient caregivers of the course of the patient's illness. This would enable the family to be prepared for the limitations that illness may impose.

Many of my reflections on illness and suffering are unorthodox because they do not always conform to our culture's views of illness. I have found my terminal illness to be empowering because I have seen it as a unique opportunity to live my life as I wish and to say what I feel needs to be said. I have come to believe Viktor Frankl's view that we can find meaning in suffering. Some, though not all, patients experience this empowerment.

My reflections on illness and suffering are also unorthodox because they are often at odds with our culture's expectations of how sick people should act. I think that if many more of us were "sick," our society would be much "healthier." To the extent that a sickness, and mainly a terminal illness, forces you to consider what is important in your life, to prioritize your time, to realize that life really matters, and to be more honest with yourself and with others, it has certainly brought you psychological health.

Because I am a nonconformist this book will reveal some of my opinions about the problems of our society. If you tend to be a conformist you may quite likely disagree with me—but this book should get you to ask some questions about the nature of our society. HCPs should remember that you will have patients that are nonconformists—so try something challenging and visualize me as your patient!

As a "sick" person, I believe that much of the savagery of our culture is related to our preoccupation with things that, in the end, may not matter. What really matters are our values and how we act upon them—what we do with our life. Our values, reflective of our spirit (or soul), are extensively discussed in chapter 5.

A NOTE TO MEDICAL STUDENTS

You are about to enter a noble profession. To be a good doctor you not only must be technologically competent but must go well beyond the "tricks of the trade." You must be able to show patients that you care whether they live—let them see your passion and your interest in their lives. This form of caring is much more than respecting them. You must provide patients encouragement and hope even in the face of suffering.

Your medical school will demand technical competence. Schools are increasingly ensuring that you be sensitive to patients: that you communicate in appropriate ways and involve patients in decisions about their care. But until medical schools require courses like "How to Love Patients," you will be on your own to figure out how to affirm, respect, comfort, and nurture them. Making health care patient-centered involves recognizing that patients are more than their physical bodies, and caring for them involves more than treating their disease but also giving attention to their psychological and spiritual needs. This book provides a holistic view of the many factors that affect a patient's health.

For good reasons, physician training piques interest in a person's disease, but it places much less emphasis on the person with the disease. As a result, a beginning medical student may be more interested in seeing patients' cancer lesions[3] than asking how they are coping with their illness and assisting them to meet the challenges (and opportunities) of terminal illness.

Patients are increasingly dissatisfied with their doctors. Some dissatisfaction can be eliminated by improving communication, by restoring trust to the physician/patient relationship, and by meeting the human needs of patients. As discussed in chapter 8, much of the trust that has historically been the foundation of the physician/patient relationship has been abrogated by financial incentives to which doctors are subject (i.e., financial incentives health maintenance organizations [HMOs] have imposed upon doctors).

This book asks you to do more conceptual thinking than medical schools will require. If doctors are filled with existential angst and do not believe that life has meaning, they surely will not see any "meaning" in suffering. And you cannot effectively communicate with patients about life and death matters unless you have thought about your own death and answered some rather philosophical questions, such as

- Where do I find meaning in my life?
- What is the nature of the contribution I will make to our society (e.g., writing your own obituary will get you to consider the nature of your contributions to your family and to society)?

- What is really important to me in life?

Patients with terminal illness often want to experience life to the fullest and realize their human potential. They may seek to further their emotional development and enter intimate relationships that involve intense honesty and sharing and caring. Sometimes the terminally ill spouse will see the emotional vacuity of his or her marriage and will seek to divorce in the hope of dating a partner who will provide the emotional intensity of a person who loves life. Terminally ill persons will often work on their human qualities, such as their values and their ability to communicate better with their friends and loved ones. Consequently, the more human you can become, the more equipped you will be to love your patients.

NOTES

1. At the time I was executive director of the agency, AIDS was really a terminal illness, but over the last several years it has come to be viewed as a chronic illness.
2. Public aid "bureaucrats" have always treated me with dignity and compassion. It is the entire public aid system that I find demeaning. And I am not so sure how public aid employees treat the truly disenfranchised, such as undocumented aliens.
3. There should be legitimate awe in the disease process, for what disease can do to the body is quite unbelievable.

Acknowledgments

No book is written without the assistance of others. I wish to thank fellow lawyer Risë Terney and her spouse, Mike Adel for generously lending me their laptop during the formative stages of the manuscript—and then my sister and brother-in-law, Mary and Shubhro Sen, for financial help to get my own computer. I wish to thank Mary Wilson, who spent many hours to copy edit the manuscript before it went to the publisher. I also thank Agnes Bacher and Molly Davison-Price, who offered their opinion as to what the book was about—helpful advice to be used in marketing.

I also wish to thank the patients, doctors, and healers who provided interviews sharing their personal stories. Many librarians assisted with this project. Warm thanks to the entire staff of the New Hartford Memorial Library (you always make it an enormous pleasure to visit the library!) for their assistance getting books on interlibrary loan and to Sarah Kovaleski, now at Northeastern University. Also generous thanks to: Gordy Schiff, M.D., for sharing with me a collection of readings (*The National Health Program Reader*) compiled by Physicians for a National Health Program and Center for a National Health Program Studies; Gene Griffin, J.D., Ph.D. for his helpful insights regarding mental health treatment in hospitals versus outpatient settings; and Joseph Palmeri for references regarding the undertreatment of pain.

1

Toward a Definition of Health, Healing, and Wholeness

INTRODUCTION: DEFINING HEALTH

Definitions of health vary among cultures and people of different ethnicities, and between doctors and patients. They incorporate many perspectives about religion, spirituality, and even diet and show that health is considered more than the absence of illness or disease.[1] Consider the following definitions of health:

- The ability to remain active and productive (Harwood, 1981, pp. 233–34; Parsons, 1972, p. 110).
- The absence of pain (Fishman, Bobo, Kosub, et al., 1993, p. 161).
- Wholeness and harmony (Harwood, 1981, pp. 144, 344).
- Nonattachment to cultural norms: For example, eccentrics are mentally and physically healthier than conformists (Weeks & James, 1995, pp. 16, 248).
- People's relationships to their surroundings (Gunderson, 1995, p. 682), including adaptation to different stresses (Helman, 1990, p. 251).
- People's relationships to their families (see ibid., p. 242): People's emotional makeup and personalities are often based on their experiences in their families of origin: the emotional traits that they develop may be the cause of their psychosomatic disorders (Minuchin, Rosman, & Baker, 1978).
- The ability to "let go" (including acceptance and detachment) (Dossey, 1995, p. 59; Berry, 1995, p. 62) and the ability to accept "what is": The ability to accept the situation forms the basis for our dedication to reality. As Scott Peck said, "Mental health is an ongoing process of dedication to reality at all costs" (Peck, 1983, p. 162).
- The ability to realize our spiritual potential ("Health is the realization of human potential when the human realizes God's kingdom 'in us' and His presence 'inside us'" [Constantelos, 1991, p. 22]).

The medical profession's focus on the alleviation or treatment of disease could be considered too narrow in light of these definitions of health. Patients, unlike physicians, see health as affected by many psychosocial factors (see Roter & Hall, 1993, p. 9), such as the ability to adapt to social, physical, and environmental changes. Increasingly, however, doctors are beginning to address these psychosocial factors (see Stewart, Brown, Weston, et al., 1995). Even medical schools are offering courses that are increasingly patient-centered and explore the social, psychological, and spiritual aspects of illness.

The definitions of health given here are quite broad. Some criticize overly broad definitions of health because they often overlap with definitions of well-being and, therefore, make health impossible to study (Antonovsky, 1979, p. 68).[2] But a comprehensive definition of health should be independent of whether the elements of the definition can be easily studied scientifically. Health is also influenced by

- the beliefs of patients and doctors (the topic of chapter 2);
- the emotions and certain personality types (the topic of chapter 4);
- the nature of healing including psychological factors that promote healing (these are discussed later);
- the individual's sense of coherence (defined later) (ibid., p. 226);
- cultural and ethnic beliefs;
- one's feeling of "community" provided by support groups and close interactions with family and friends;
- one's social class and educational level (Shweder, 1997; Tyroler, 1983);
- life events, such as the death of close family members (Murphy & Brown, 1980); and
- job dissatisfaction (see *Work in America*, 1973), which also measures our ability to get along with others and to communicate and cooperate with them.

The Beliefs of Patients and Doctors

Because most patients strongly believe that medications will either treat or cure their condition, these beliefs create a positive physiological effect, even if these patients are given a placebo or sugar pill. Conversely, patients' negative beliefs may adversely affect their health. Patients who express fear that they will die during surgery frequently do (Hackett & Weisman, 1961).

Doctors' beliefs ultimately influence their patients' responses to treatment. Doctors' enthusiasm about the drugs they prescribe also affects patient responses to them (Benson with Stark, 1996, p. 34). Because many doctors seem to be highly enthusiastic about newly released drugs, patients often show improvement in their condition at the time these drugs are given, even when future data on the drug indicates it is ineffective in treating particular conditions.

Emotions and Certain Personality Types

The onset or aggravation of disease is affected by the emotions. Diabetes, for example, can get out of control during personal crises (Slawson, Flynn, &

Kollar, 1963). When emotions such as grief or fear are extreme, people may experience increased morbidity and mortality, presumably due to a mechanism that overwhelms the autonomic nervous system (Lynch, 1985; Alexander, French, & Pollock, 1968). Psychosomatic disease may be related to psychological conflict in childhood, as in persons with hypertension who learned as children to repress anger because they feared losing the affection of others (Alexander, French, & Pollock, 1968, p. 20).

Psychological Factors That Promote Healing

Healing is promoted by optimism and a positive attitude. As discussed in chapter 4, optimistic men who were followed for eight years after their first heart attack had greater survival rates than pessimistic men (Peterson, Maier, & Seligman, 1993). Healing is also promoted by maintaining hope and by having purpose and meaning in life.

Chapter 4 also considers the relationship of control over one's environment to survival. One researcher has observed that nursing home residents felt "less helpless when they were given a sense of responsibility for themselves" (Langer, 1983, p. 101). This responsibility may only include a simple act like watering a plant on a regular basis. Eighteen months later, only half as many subjects had died in the responsibility-induced group as in the control group (ibid.). And workers in low control jobs have a statistically significant and increased risk of dying from cardiovascular disease than workers in high control jobs with a great deal of job-related autonomy (Johnson, Stewart, & Hall, 1996).

Since people are social, it is not surprising that intimate relationships, or relationships in which there is honest and open dialogue, also promote healing. Because of the honest communication in support groups, it might not be surprising that women with metastatic breast cancer participating in such groups survived twice as long as women who merely received standard medical treatment for their cancer (Spiegel, Bloom, Kraemer, et al., 1989). Last, as discussed in many of the chapters, acceptance of one's illness may not only be important for the development of peace of mind, but has been considered a reason for healing.

Maintenance of Cultural Stability and Norms

When people are removed from their culture, as occurs with emigration, they often become ill. For example, when Native Americans move from reservations to urban centers, they often experience increased blood pressure (DeStefano, Coulehan, & Wiant, 1979; Braxton, 1970). Removal from their culture is believed to be the basis for the "sudden" death of Hmong refugees (Benson with Stark, 1996, pp. 84–86).

The Patient's Educational Level and Social Class

Some studies have shown that educational level is significantly related to patient mortality rates (Tyroler, 1983).[3] In one study of 2094 males aged 30–69 with mild hypertension, the risk of dying was significantly higher among whites with less education; for blacks, there was a sevenfold increase in death rate among those with the least education.[4]

Many studies also suggest an association between social class and illness (Shweder, 1997; Syme & Berkman, 1976), independent of the wealthy's better access to health care,[5] the poor's hazardous work or living conditions, and life-style differences between rich and poor (ibid.). However, the reason for the association between social class and illness is not fully understood. Consider some of the following evidence (and theories) to support this association:

- Poorer and less educated people are more likely to smoke (Pear, 1993).
- Many social ills associated with poverty often become medical problems ("U.S. Social Ills Become Medical Problems," 1992). These social ills include the breakdown of the family structure, chronic underemployment, homelessness, violence, and even despair (ibid.). The decreased social health of children and youth has been attributed to increases in child abuse, teenage suicide, drug abuse, and the high school dropout rate (Ravo, 1996).
- People with tuberculosis and schizophrenia, persons who are alcoholics, and persons who are victims of multiple accidents and suicides have a marginal status in society (Cassel, 1974). They have been deprived of meaningful social contact (ibid.). A "social-network index" has been used to show that the morbidity and mortality in the lower classes were associated with their "questionable ability to maintain enduring and effective social ties" (Syme & Berkman, 1976, p. 2).
- The environment in which the poor reside is depleted of social capital ("the features of social organization, such as civil participation, norms of reciprocity and trust in others, that facilitate cooperation for mutual benefit") (Kawachi, Kennedy, Lochner, et al., 1997).
- Rising income inequality results in increased levels of frustration, which adversely affect behavior and health (see ibid.).

The Individual's Sense of Coherence

Antonovsky believes that the stronger the sense of coherence of individuals and groups, "the more adequately will they cope with the stressors imminent in life, and the more likely are they to maintain or improve their positions on the health/disease continuum" (Antonovsky, 1979, p. 226). He defines coherence as

a global orientation that expresses the extent to which one has a pervasive, enduring though dynamic feeling of confidence that one's internal and external environments are predictable and that there is a high probability that things will work out as well as can be reasonably expected. (ibid., p. 123)

CONCEPTIONS ABOUT WHOLENESS

The word *health* is derived from "wholeness" (Gunderson, 1995, p. 680). The concept of wholeness implies that one can be "whole" despite being ill—admittedly, this characterization would not make sense to most Americans. Oddly enough, Rabbi Harold Kushner has said that "in some strange sense, we are more whole when we are incomplete, when we are missing something" (Kushner, 1996, p. 179). Kushner suggests that when we are incomplete, we strive to achieve wholeness and to become more complete.[6] To be whole, therefore, means to

- have mental health or "peace of mind" despite illness;
- strive to remain productive despite the limitations imposed by illness;
- live life to the "fullest" and experience the full range of emotions and moods (from happiness to sadness). It means to live in spite of illness and to find meaning in life in spite of tragedy; as discussed in chapter 3, psychiatrist Viktor Frankl, who survived internment in three different Nazi concentration camps, has noted that it is possible to find meaning in suffering (see Frankl, 1957, pp. 122 et seq. [chapter 2]).
- adapt to life's challenges;
- be able to be generous and give of oneself without feeling diminished (see Kushner, 1996, p. 179);
- accept one's limitations and let go of unrealistic dreams without feeling like a failure for doing so (ibid.);
- be in harmony with one's environment.

Developing Peace of Mind Despite Illness

Despite illness you can acquire a positive mental attitude and/or peace of mind. You can learn to choose your attitude and to "control" your experience, that is by controlling your thoughts about your experience. Viktor E. Frankl recalled that concentration camp survivors

can remember the men who walked through the huts comforting others, giving away their last piece of bread. They may have been few in number, but they offer sufficient proof that everything can be taken away from a person but one thing: the last of the human freedoms—to choose one's attitude in any given set of circumstances. (Frankl, 1963, p. 104)

Living Life to the Fullest

As discussed more fully in chapter 3, when we live life to the fullest we do the following:

- Focus on relationships and make them deeper and richer: to do this we must be more honest and we must make ourselves vulnerable.

- Connect with others as human beings: this may require us to listen to them more carefully and to be more attentive to and interested in their journeys.
- Grapple with pain, suffering, and tragedy, not ignoring it and failing to deal with it.
- Live in the moment and appreciate our present experiences.

Adapting to Life's Challenges

When we adapt to life's challenges we are not devastated by failure but strengthened by it. We learn to take things in stride and to accept that we cannot always realize our dreams when we would like. In short, we must be flexible enough to make room for setbacks.

Being in Harmony with One's Environment

The concept of wholeness is integral to notions of harmony. For example, to be whole we must be in harmony with the following:

- Our mind and spirit. This is the Chinese and Navaho view of health (Harwood, 1981, pp. 144, 344).
- Our surroundings (Gunderson, 1995). In certain circumstances, patients may heal faster at home than in the hospital. In a British study of 350 randomly chosen coronary patients, the death rate for those in intensive care units was higher than for those convalescing at home (Ferguson, 1980, pp. 244–45). Being aware that patients may react differently to their surroundings is the basis for recognizing the need to understand patients' life circumstances (like the stress patients are under) in order to treat their illnesses (note: the effects of stress are further discussed in chapter 4).

CONCEPTIONS ABOUT HEALING

Introduction

The concept of being healed is distinct from being cured of one's condition. Christiane Northrup, a former president of the American Holistic Medical Association, has said that "you can heal your life but have a sick body" (Dossey, 1995, p. 58). In order for a person to heal, several have said that one must

- have a passion for living (ibid., p. 56 [view of Jeanne Achterberg]). This view is closely related to that of Viktor Frankl, who developed a form of psychotherapy to assist patients to find meaning in their lives. Frankl suggested that people who have meaning in their lives may live longer than those without it (see the discussion in chapter 3).
- let go of one's concerns about the self and the ego (ibid., p. 59). Many have talked about the meaning and purpose that may come into our lives when we "serve others"

(Benson with Stark, 1996, p. 181; Luks, 1992). This is, of course, one way to deflect the focus off ourselves.

- accept our circumstances, including our illnesses. With such acceptance we are often able to be transformed by our illnesses. This acceptance may also give us peace of mind and allow us to focus on and appreciate what we have.
- experience love in one's life (see LeShan, 1974).
- have support from the members of one's community (Berry, 1995).

Almost all of the factors listed involve being empty: the quality people have when they are filled with gratitude and acceptance (Dossey, 1991, p. 199). Being empty implies that we are open to possibilities everywhere (from our work to our family life) and that we set aside our "agendas" and preconceived expectations. For example, if we invite someone to dinner we might expect to discuss particular topics or issues, but in a state of being "empty," we set aside our expectations and let the evening's conversation take its own course. When we are "empty" we do not exert our will, often under the influence of our ego, upon others.

Having a Passion for Living

> The moment a man questions the meaning and value of life he is sick.
> Sigmund Freud, in a letter to Princess Bonaparte,
> quoted in Frankl,
> *The Will to Meaning*, p. 87

To have a passion for living, one must enjoy one's daily activities and work; be invested in, involved in, and enthusiastic about one's work; be enriched by one's relationships with others. We cannot be passionate about living unless we do what we want to do.

Frankl believed that man's ultimate search in life is to find meaning. And Freud too suggested that persons without meaning in their lives are sick. The search for meaning is akin to a spiritual striving.

Others have equated a passion for living with a religious dimension. Kelsey believes that without faith "the soul despairs and gives up the struggle for life" (Kelsey, 1995, p. 303). Those who give up this struggle do not have a passion for living.

We can also "heal into death" (Siegel, 1993, p. 175). This definition of healing assumes that dying persons may resolve major life issues (ibid.) such as repairing damaged relationships. To do such things is to remain involved with life. Consequently, it is not ironic that one can remain passionate about living while "healing into death."

What it means to "live" is not an easy question to answer and one that cannot be answered with universal agreement. How have some contemporary thinkers answered this question?

- Eleanor Roosevelt suggested that to live life, we must "taste experience to the utmost [and] reach out eagerly and without fear for newer and richer experience" (Roosevelt, 1960, p. xii). She believed that "what keeps our interest in life and makes us look forward to tomorrow is giving pleasure to other people" (ibid., p. 95).
- Erich Fromm said that the person who loves life "prefers to construct rather than to retain. He is capable of wondering, and he prefers to see something new to the security of finding confirmation of the old. He loves the adventure of living more than he does certainty" (Fromm, 1964, p. 47). Fromm also said that for love of life to develop, persons must have "the freedom to create and to construct, to wonder and to venture" (ibid., p. 52) and that such freedom requires individuals to be "active and responsible" (ibid.).
- Viktor Frankl said that "[l]ife ultimately means taking the responsibility to find the right answer to its problems and to fulfill the tasks which it constantly sets for each individual" (Frankl, 1963, p. 122).

Letting Go of Our Concerns about the Self and Our Preoccupation with Illness

Although the service of others deflects our focus off ourselves, one of its by-products may be happiness (see Luks, 1992). The great physician and humanitarian Albert Schweitzer said that "[t]he only ones among you who will be really happy are those who will have sought and found how to serve" (Bryant, 1991, p. 150).

Accepting Our Circumstances

It is important for ill people to accept their illnesses:

- Navaho medicine woman Annie Kahn says that "to heal, one must . . . accept." This very act causes healing (Perone, Stockel, & Krueger, 1989, p. 36).
- Carl Jung said that we cannot change anything unless we accept it (Siegel, 1993, p. 24).

By accepting our illnesses we are able to

- look to the future and develop tasks and strategies to realize our goals (by looking to the future we become hopeful). Cancer surgeon Bernie Siegel has reminded us that acceptance is not resignation (Siegel, 1986, p. 177);
- focus on the things we can change: Although we cannot change the presence of disease in our bodies, we can change our attitudes about our disease;
- stop grieving for what we have lost—the bodily functions that our illness may have taken from us—and focus upon what we have and are able to continue to do. We might also focus upon what we have "gained" from the illness or what the illness has taught us.

Some studies have shown that spiritual devotion and acceptance in some individuals with cancer preceded their cure of cancer (Dossey, 1993, p. 31). Such individuals may have stopped hoping for being cured of cancer, but that is far different from giving up on life or failing to be "involved with life."

In the American tradition, acceptance is not a natural state. Our culture does everything possible to encourage persons to deny their death: it is not death-embracing but death-avoiding. Some people may live under the illusion that with the proper diet and exercise they will escape the certainty of death.

Although it is probably difficult to envision oneself on one's deathbed, there are many ways to think constructively about one's mortality. When we are fully aware that we will eventually die, we often take steps to lead a more fulfilled or rich life.

In the West, facing death is made difficult by our culture's aversion to both "uncertainty" and solitude. Our aversion to uncertainty is illustrated by our discomfort when doctors cannot predict whether our illnesses will be "cured" despite our treatment. Our aversion to solitude, a method to reflect and examine the nature of our life, is probably the result of cultural norms that do not value inner peace (Benson with Stark, 1996, p. 263); imply that to be valuable we must be "busy"; and cause others to believe that to be happy we must possess various goods and products. Consequently, the consumerism of our culture militates against our having ample time for moments of solitude.

Receiving Support from the Members of Our Community

Human beings have an intrinsic need to interact with others—they are social beings. When we are community-deprived, we feel isolated. The adverse health consequences of social and physical isolation cannot be overemphasized. The positive consequences of being a member of a community—such as occurs when people enter support groups—have been extensively studied (Spiegel, Bloom, Kraemer, et al., 1989).

Sources of Healing

Patients can heal their bodies and minds in many ways. When patients attempt to heal their bodies, they often consult either nontraditional (e.g., herbalists,[7] acupuncturists) or traditional (e.g., physicians) healers. And, as discussed later, our own bodies possess an intrinsic capacity to heal. But health also has "mental components." When it comes to maintaining mental health, we must remember that patients also consult a variety of nontraditional (e.g., spiritists,[8] cuandero[9]) and traditional (e.g., psychiatrists, social workers, clergy) "healers."

As discussed throughout this book, we can do a great deal to preserve our own mental health. We can take steps to enhance our peace of mind and take control of certain aspects of our lives (i.e., by communicating more honestly with others).

The Healer Within. Many have written about the body's intrinsic capacity to heal (see Justice, 1987, pp. 309 et seq.; Weil, 1995, p. 71). Some believe that man's ability to survive, an ability that predated antibiotics and even surgery, is evidence for internal healing mechanisms (Weil, 1995, p. 71). Scientific evidence of the body's internal healing mechanisms is that cells have receptors to which antibiotics can attach. This implies that the body must have endogenous antibiotics to fight infection.

As discussed in chapter 5, even the unconscious mind is believed to promote healing. Dream analysts have reported that the dreams of demented persons made "sense" (Muff, 1996). One implication of such a study is that, since the psyche remains aware of the "larger issues," it is attempting to preserve the body's natural and "healed" state. And the fact that people's dreams may give them "clues" to suggest that they are suffering from a physical illness (Donnelly & McPeak, 1996) is another indication that the body's "warning" or "alarm" system is aimed to preserve a state of homeostasis.

Those concerned about the existence of any internal healing system are also concerned with ways to stimulate it (Weil, 1995). Many believe that self-healing mechanisms are mobilized when persons perceive a sense of control (Justice, 1987, p. 309).

Nontraditional Forms of Healing. Many patients seek treatment outside hospitals, clinics, and doctors' offices. Patients often treat themselves at home and seek alternative treatments from nontraditional healers. Studies estimate that between 70 and 90 percent of all "illness episodes" are treated outside mainstream medical facilities either at home or by alternative healers (Harwood, 1981, p. 25).

Those who seek nontraditional treatments come from different social classes. Whereas many poor Hispanics may consult folk healers and others healers, discussed later, studies of Anglos who seek nontraditional healing indicate that they are better educated and better-off financially than nonusers of alternative practices (Blais, Maïga, & Aboubacar, 1997; Eisenberg, Kessler, Foster, et al., 1993).[10]

There are many reasons why patients consult nontraditional healers, often before seeking traditional treatments. In many cultures, mental health problems are stigmatizing (Shum, 1996 [Asian Americans]; Qureshi, 1989 [Indians]). Consequently, some ethnic clients will go to nontraditional healers who are also members of their own ethnic group to cope better with such stigma.

Health professionals should realize that they typically see only a select group of patients: those sick enough to require acute care in hospitals or those who seek regular care in physician's offices. Health professionals may not realize that for every acutely ill person with a particular disease they treat in the hospital, there may be hundreds or thousands of persons with that same disease who are functioning quite well with that same disease in the community.

HOW DIFFERENT CULTURES VIEW DEATH

In many cultures, thinking about death is embraced. This often occurs, for example, in cultures with a large number of practicing Buddhists and Hindus. In Hindu India, it is said that persons are preoccupied with eternity (Darian, 1988, p. xiii). Buddhist practices are often aimed at reducing or eliminating the deleterious effects of the ego and the focus on or preoccupation with things that involve the self: the things that make us feel better than, or more special than, another. These include appearance, status, money, and even health. Apparently, the Buddha recommended meditation on death "as a corrective for persons in whom greed and attachment predominate" (Ramaswami & Sheikh, 1989, p. 118). The Buddhist concept of detachment is of course a reminder that we should not be too attached to "things" because they are impermanent and will inevitably cause suffering. This suffering may arise from jealousy and greed, negative emotions evoked when we compare ourselves to others and covet their possessions.

The gradual or complete acceptance of death may involve muting or "killing" the ego and the feeling that we can direct our destiny.

In Indian society, which is predominantly Hindu, death is spoken about more openly than in the United States and people may be heard to say that they are ready to "welcome" death at any time (Vatuk, 1996, p. 127). In the Hindu view, "the sudden, painless death of an elderly person is not regarded as a fortunate one" because such a person had no time to prepare for this critical passage (ibid., p. 123). "The ultimate and critical sign of the good life is measured by how a person attains his death" (ibid. quoting Madan, 1988, p. 122). In preparing for death, the elderly may take leave of their family and friends (ibid., p. 123), or even go to the city of Banaras, for it is believed that the souls of those who die there will be liberated or released and, therefore, will not need to undergo a cycle of rebirths (ibid.).

TOWARD DEFINING PATIENT-CENTERED HEALTH CARE

Patient-centered health care focuses on the *patient's goals and expectations* (i.e., those regarding treatment and treatment alternatives) and is delivered in a *holistic manner* with *utmost compassion*. Patient-centered health care is holistic: health care professionals must not only be sensitive to the patient's mind/body/spirit but aware of how the patient's environment (e.g., support networks) affect the patient's health. Patients also have every right to expect that

**EFFORTS BY HOSPITALS TO PRODUCE
PATIENT-CENTERED CARE**

Some hospitals have instituted programs that are sensitive to the unique and particular needs of patients. St. Mary's Hospital and Health Center (Tucson, Arizona) began its "traditional Indian Medical Program" in 1984 after one Apache nurse pointed out to the staff that Native Americans were not given the spiritual support they needed or that their beliefs were not given the respect that they deserved (Allshouse, 1993, p. 27). Now, on request, Native American patients can receive a medicine man's spiritual counseling and prayer services. Other traditional healers are also welcomed and any ceremonies performed are not interfered with.

Many patients have complained that the rules and procedures of the hospital bureaucracy serve the interests of the latter and not of patients. Planetree Model Hospital Unit at California Pacific Medical Center tries to accommodate patients by scheduling tests at times convenient for patients. Furthermore, at the Cooperative Care Unit of the New York University Medical Center (New York, New York) patients' meals are served in a cafeteria where patients can select from different types of food, allowing them a choice in the meals they eat as well as the time at which they eat. Patients on this unit are also allowed to wear "street clothes," although they must wear identification badges.

their physicians will be both technically competent and compassionate. They should be able to feel that it matters to their doctor whether they live or die.

The role of caring and compassion for both nurses and physicians is being extensively discussed in medical literature (Benner & Wrubel, 1989; Gaut & Leininger, 1991; Mayerhoff, 1971). Although this topic is extensively discussed in chapter 5, it is important to recognize that, in the West, medicine became "secularized" and less attentive to needs of the patient's spirit. Of particular interest is that in parts of the East—and particularly in Tibet—monks are also physicians (see chapter 5, where the views of a prominent Tibetan monk-physician are discussed).

To produce patient-centered health care, physicians and hospital personnel will need to change how they view and interact with patients. Some medical personnel attempt to enforce rules that are aimed at their own convenience and do not necessarily consider the interests of the patient. Changes at the hospital level might be more difficult to implement merely because it seems more daunting to change a bureaucratic organization than an individual. But some hospitals have implemented such changes.

Physicians can significantly contribute to our health. But they must appreciate the many psychosocial and spiritual issues that impact upon patients' health and understand that any definition of health must incorporate the concept of wholeness. This broader view of health will lead to some new roles for physicians (see particularly chapter 8). These new roles may include some of the following:

- Doctors will have to get to know both their patients and patients' families and the support networks they might use in order to understand, counsel, and treat patients more effectively.
- Physicians may need to be better advocates for patients. To be an advocate is to show respect for patients, such that patients feel that doctors care whether they live or die. This advocacy role may take doctors out of the examining room and into the legislature, where important policies affecting patients' welfare are made.
- Many patients expect that medical professionals will address their spiritual needs (Benson with Stark, 1996, p. 121) because the spiritual quality of life is often more important to them than the physical reality. This expectation has led to many patients' desire that their physicians not only pray for them but with them (Dossey, 1996, p. 69).

CHAPTER SUMMARY

Definitions of health vary among cultures, among people of different ethnicities, and between doctors and patients. Many definitions go beyond the biomedical definition that health is merely the absence of disease; they incorporate religious, psychological, and social perspectives. Health is also influenced by many social parameters such as our feelings of "community," social class and educational level, and satisfaction with our jobs. Health is also profoundly influenced by patients' and doctors' beliefs and by emotions. For example, sudden death has accompanied people facing incredible fear or loss (e.g., death of a spouse). Patients of different ethnicities "construct" illnesses, known as folk illnesses, and as a result they may seek the expertise of nontraditional healers, because these illnesses are not recognized by traditional medicine.

Both traditional and nontraditional healers may exert an influence over their patients far beyond the effect of any substances (e.g., herbs or drugs) that they may prescribe. This influence may have psychological and/or spiritual roots and may involve counseling, inspiring, and/or offering patients support, understanding, or hope. Because many cuanderos or folk healers in the Latin tradition are insightful into the acculturation pressures and stresses upon immigrants, they are in a position to counsel patients so that they can develop peace of mind. And as discussed in chapter 6, the role of many traditional healers, such as physicians, should be to offer patients hope continually.

This book proposes an expanded role for physicians, one premised on the notion that for doctors to get beyond being mere technicians and to practice the art of medicine, they must be more attentive to caring for patients. According to patients, this role should even include praying with patients in order to meet their spiritual needs.

The terms *healing* and *wholeness* are frequently encountered in discussions about health and wellness. Although they have been defined differently, these two concepts are virtually synonymous, for to be healed is also to be whole. Both concepts involve acceptance of one's condition. With acceptance, peace of mind inevitably follows.

NOTES

1. The meaning of the word *illness* is distinguished from that of the word *disease*: the former is what you feel and the latter is what you have (Barsky, 1988, p. 37).

2. Antonovsky is critical of the World Health Organization's definition of health, that is, that *health* is "a state of complete physical, mental, and social well-being and not merely the absence of disease or infirmity" (Antonovsky, 1979, p. 52). He implies that this definition makes health impossible to study because it "declares flatly that everything people feel about their state of well-being is part of health" (ibid., p. 53).

3. Mortality rate typically reflects deaths from violence, accidents, occupational injuries, and diseases (see Pear, 1993).

4. The differences in mortality rates for blacks and whites remain substantial regardless of social class. One study reported that black men were at least *twice as likely to die prematurely as white men within each social class studied* (emphasis added) (Barnett, Armstrong, & Casper, 1997).

5. A Rand Corporation study of almost 4,000 poor people supports this point of view. The study concluded that free health care did not improve the health status of poor people (Kolata, 1993).

6. Kushner believes that "[t]he man who has everything is in some ways a poor man. He will never know what it feels like to yearn, to hope, to nourish his soul with the dream of something better. He will never know the experience of having someone who loves him give him something he has always wanted and never had" (Kushner, 1996, p. 179).

7. Many herbs in the Hispanic community are purchased in stores known as *botánicas*. Botánicas are patronized for nervous, digestive, respiratory, rheumatic, and sometimes genitourinary conditions (Harwood, 1981, p. 446). It seems that some of the herbs prescribed at botánicas may be harmful (e.g., wormwood, mugwort, laurel, bloodroot) (ibid., p. 447).

8. Spiritism posits that we are surrounded by an invisible world of good and evil spirits that may penetrate this world to influence human lives. Persons who have gained "psychic faculties" over the spirits are often sought as folk healers to cure emotional problems, particularly in the Puerto Rican culture (Rogler & Hollingshead, 1985).

9. Cuanderos are folk healers in the Latin tradition. Apparently, at least for Puerto Ricans, cuanderos are "little used today" (Harwood, 1981, p. 448). The curing power of cuanderos is attributed to divinely bestowed powers (ibid., p. 310). Studies have shown that cuanderos are "good intuitive psychologists who display considerable insight into both intracultural and acculturation pressures and stresses" (ibid., p. 311).

10. Some of the forms of alternative medicine are the following: relaxation techniques, chiropractic, massage, imagery, spiritual healing, weight-loss programs, life-style diets (e.g., macrobiotic), megavitamins, self-help groups, energy healing, biofeedback, hypnosis, homeopathy, acupuncture, and folk remedies (Eisenberg, Kessler, Foster, et al., 1993).

SUGGESTED READING

Harwood, Alan, ed. *Ethnicity and Medical Care*. Cambridge, MA: Harvard University Press, 1981.

REFERENCES

Alexander, Franz, Thomas M. French, and George H. Pollock. *Psychosomatic Specificity*. Chicago, IL: University of Chicago Press, 1968.

Allshouse, Kimberly D. "Treating Patients as Individuals." In *Through the Patient's Eyes: Understanding and Promoting Patient-Centered Care*. M. Gerteis, S. Edgman-Levitan, J. Daley, et al., eds. San Francisco: Jossey-Bass, 1993, pp. 19–44.

Antonovsky, Aaron. *Health, Stress and Coping*. San Francisco: Jossey-Bass, 1979.

Barnett, Elizabeth, Donna Armstrong, and Michele Casper. "Social Class and Premature Mortality among Men: A Method for State-Based Surveillance." 87 *American Journal of Public Health* 1521–25 (Sept. 1997).

Barsky, Arthur J. *Worried Sick: Our Troubled Quest for Wellness*. Boston: Little, Brown, 1988.

Benner, Patricia E., and Judith Wrubel. *The Primacy of Caring: Stress and Coping in Health and Illness*. Menlo Park, CA: Addison-Wesley, 1989.

Benson, Herbert, with Marg Stark. *Timeless Healing: The Power and Biology of Belief*. New York: Scribner, 1996.

Berry, Wendell. "Health Is Membership: The Community Is the Smallest Unit of Health." *Utne Reader* 60–63 (Sept./Oct. 1995).

Blais, Régis, Aboubacrine Maïga, and Alarou Aboubacar. "How Different Are Users and Non-Users of Alternative Medicine?" 88 *Canadian Journal of Public Health* 159–62 (May/June 1997).

Braxton, M. Alfred. "Blood Pressure Changes among Male Navaho Migrants to an Urban Environment." 7 *The Canadian Review of Sociology and Anthropology* 189–200 (1970).

Bryant, Roberta Jean. *Stop Improving Yourself and Start Living*. San Rafael, CA: New World Library, 1991.

Cassel, John. "Psychosocial Processes and 'Stress': Theoretical Formulation." 4 *International Journal of Health Services* 471–82 (1974).

Constantelos, Demetrios J. "The Interface of Medicine and Religion." In *Health and Faith: Medical, Psychological and Religious Dimensions*. J. T. Chirban, ed. Lanham, MD: University Press of America, 1991, pp. 13–24.

Darian, Steven. *A Ganges of the Mind: A Journey on the River of Dreams*. Delhi, India: Ratna Sagar, 1988.

DeStefano, Frank, John L. Coulehan, and M. Kenneth Wiant. "Blood Pressure Survey on the Navajo Indian Reservation." 109 *American Journal of Epidemiology* 335–45 (1979).

Donnelly, Gloria F., and Concetta DeLuca McPeak. "Dreams: Their Function in Health and Illness." 10 *Holistic Nursing Practice* 61–68 (July 1996).

Dossey, Larry. "Healing Happens: The Miracle of Distant Healing." *Utne Reader* 51–59 (Sept./Oct. 1995).

———. *Healing Words: The Power of Prayer and the Practice of Medicine*. San Francisco: HarperSan Francisco, 1993.

———. *Meaning and Medicine: A Doctor's Tales of Breakthrough and Healing*. New York: Bantam, 1991.

———. *Prayer Is Good Medicine*. New York: HarperCollins, 1996.

Eisenberg, David, Ronald C. Kessler, Cindy Foster, et al. "Unconventional Medicine in the United States: Prevalence, Costs, and Patterns of Use." 328 *New England Journal of Medicine* 246–52 (Jan. 28, 1993).

Ferguson, Marilyn. *The Aquarian Conspiracy: Personal and Social Transformation for*

Our Time. New York: G. P. Putnam, 1980.

Fishman, Barbara M., Loretta Bobo, Kristy Kosub, et al. "Cultural Issues in Serving Minority Populations: Emphasis on Mexican Americans and African Americans." 306 *American Journal of Medical Sciences* 160–66 (Sept. 1993).

Frankl, Viktor E. *The Doctor and the Soul: An Introduction to Logotherapy*. New York: Alfred A. Knopf, 1957.

———. *Man's Search for Meaning: An Introduction to Logotherapy*. New York: Pocket Books, 1963.

———. *The Will to Meaning: Foundation and Applications of Logotherapy*. New York and Cleveland: New American Library and World Publishing, 1969.

Fromm, Erich. *The Heart of Man: Its Genius for Good and Evil*. New York: Harper & Row, 1964.

Gaut, Delores A., and Madeleine M. Leininger, eds. *Caring: The Compassionate Healer*. New York: National League for Nursing Press, 1991.

Gunderson, Richard B. "Rethinking Our Basic Concepts of Health and Disease." 70 *Academic Medicine* 676–83 (Aug. 1995).

Hackett, Thomas P., and Avery D. Weisman. "Predilection to Death: Death and Dying as a Psychiatric Problem." 23 *Psychosomatic Medicine* 232–56 (1961).

Harwood, Alan, ed. *Ethnicity and Medical Care*. Cambridge, MA: Harvard University Press, 1981.

Helman, Cecil G. *Culture, Health and Illness: An Introduction for Health Professionals*, 2nd ed. London: Butterworth, 1990.

Johnson, Jeffrey V., Walter Stewart, and Ellen M. Hall. "Long-Term Psychosocial Work Environment and Cardiovascular Mortality among Swedish Men." 86 *American Journal of Public Health* 324–31 (March 1996).

Justice, Blair. *Who Gets Sick: Thinking and Health*. Houston: Peak Press, 1987.

Kawachi, Ichiro, Bruce P. Kennedy, Kimberly Lochner, et al. "Social Capital, Income Inequality and Mortality." 87 *American Journal of Public Health* 1491–98 (Sept. 1997).

Kelsey, Morton. *Healing and Christianity*, 3rd ed. Minneapolis: Augsberg Fortress, 1995.

Kolata, Gina. "Will U.S. Be Healthier? Maybe Not, Experts Say National Studies Show That People Do Not Become Healthier Because They Go to Doctors." *N.Y. Times*, Oct. 17, 1993, Sec. 1, p. 1.

Kushner, Harold S. *How Good Do We Have to Be? A New Understanding of Guilt and Forgiveness*. Boston: Little, Brown, 1996.

Langer, Ellen. *The Psychology of Control*. Beverly Hills, CA: Sage Publications, 1983.

LeShan, Lawrence. *The Medium, The Mystic, and the Physicist: Toward a General Theory of the Paranormal*. New York: Viking Press, 1974.

Luks, Allan. *The Healing Power of Doing Good: The Health and Spiritual Benefits of Helping Others*. New York: Fawcett Columbine, 1992.

Lynch, James J. *The Language of the Heart: The Body's Response to Human Dialogue*. New York: Basic Books, 1985.

Madan, T.N. *Non-Renunciation: Themes and Interpretations of Hindu Culture*. Delhi: Oxford University Press, 1988.

Mayerhoff, Milton. *On Caring*. New York: Harper & Row, 1971.

Minuchin, Salvador, Bernice L. Rosman, and Lester Baker. *Psychosomatic Families: Anorexia Nervosa in Context*. Cambridge, MA: Harvard University Press, 1978.

Muff, Janet. "From the Wings of Night: Dream Work with Persons Who Have Acquired Immunodeficiency Syndrome." 10 *Holistic Nursing Practice* 69–87 (1996).

Murphy, Elaine, and George W. Brown. "Life Events, Psychiatric Disturbance and

Physical Illness." 136 *British Journal of Psychiatry* 326–38 (1980).

Parsons, Talcott. "Definitions of Health and Illness in the Light of American Values and Social Structure." In *Patients, Physicians and Illness*. E.G. Jaco, ed. New York: The Free Press, 1972, pp. 107–27.

Pear, Robert. "Big Health Gap, Tied to Income, Is Found in U.S." *N.Y. Times*, July 8, 1993, Sec. A, p. 1.

Peck, M. Scott. *People of the Lie: The Hope for Healing Human Evil*. New York: Simon & Schuster, 1983.

Perone, Bobette, H. Henrietta Stockel, and Victoria Krueger. *Medicine Women, Cuanderas, and Women Doctors*. Norman, OK: University of Oklahoma Press, 1989.

Peterson, Christopher, Steven F. Maier, and Martin E.P. Seligman. *Learned Helplessness: A Theory for the Age of Personal Control*. New York: Oxford University Press, 1993.

Qureshi, Bashir. *Transcultural Medicine: Dealing with Patients from Different Cultures*. London: Kluwer Academic Publishers, 1989.

Ramaswami, Sundar, and Anees A. Sheikh. "Buddhist Psychology: Implications for Healing." In *Eastern and Western Approaches to Healing: Ancient Wisdom and Modern Knowledge*. A.A. Sheikh and K.S. Sheikh, eds. New York: Wiley, 1989, pp. 91–123.

Ravo, Nick. "25-Year Low in a Measure of Well-Being." *N.Y. Times*, Oct. 14, 1996, Sec. A, p. 11.

Rogler, Lloyd H., and August B. Hollingshead. *Trapped: Families and Schizophrenia*, 3rd ed. Maplewood, NJ: Waterfront Press, 1985.

Roosevelt, Eleanor. *You Learn by Living*. New York: Harper & Row, 1960.

Roter, Debra L., and Judith A. Hall. *Doctors Talking with Patients/Patients Talking with Doctors: Improving Communication in Medical Visits*. Westport, CT: Auburn House, 1993.

Shum, Linda May. "Asian-American Women: Cultural and Mental Health Issues." 789 *Annals of the New York Academy of Sciences* 181–90 (June 1996).

Shweder, Richard A. "It's Called Poor Health for a Reason." *N.Y. Times*, March 9, 1997, Sec. 4 (Week in Review), p. 5, col. 1.

Siegel, Bernie S. *How to Live Between Office Visits: A Guide to Life, Love and Health*. New York: HarperCollins, 1993.

————. *Love, Medicine and Miracles: Lessons Learned about Self-Healing from a Surgeon's Experience with Exceptional Patients*. New York: Harper & Row, 1986.

Slawson, Paul F., William R. Flynn, and Edward J. Kollar. "Psychological Factors Associated with the Onset of Diabetes Mellitus." 185 *Journal of the American Medical Association* 166–70 (July 20, 1963).

Spiegel, David, Joan R. Bloom, Helena C. Kraemer, et al. "Effects of Psychosocial Treatment on Survival of Patients with Metastatic Breast Cancer." *Lancet* 888–91 (Oct. 15, 1989).

Stewart, Moira, Judith Belle Brown, W. Wayne Weston, et al. *Patient-Centered Medicine: Transforming the Clinical Method*. Thousand Oaks, CA: Sage Publications, 1995.

Syme, S. Leonard, and Lisa F. Berkman. "Social Class, Susceptibility and Sickness." 104 *American Journal of Epidemiology* 1–8 (1976).

Tyroler, H.A. "Race, Education and 5-Year Mortality in HDFP Stratum 1 Referred-Care Males." In *Mild Hypertension: Recent Advances*. F. Gross and T. Strasser, eds. New York: Raven Press, 1983, pp. 163–75.

"U.S. Social Ills Become Medical Problems." *N.Y. Times*, July 2, 1992, Sec. A, p. 18.

Vatuk, Sylvia. "The Art of Dying in Hindu India." In *Facing Death: Where Culture, Religion and Medicine Meet.* H.M. Spiro, M.G. Curnen, and L.P. Wandel, eds. New Haven, CT: Yale University Press, 1996, pp. 121–28.

Weeks, David Joseph, and Jamie James. *Eccentrics: A Study of Sanity and Strangeness.* New York: Villard, 1995.

Weil, Andrew. *Spontaneous Healing: How to Discover and Enhance Your Body's Natural Ability to Maintain and Heal Itself.* New York: Alfred A. Knopf, 1995.

Work in America: Report of a Special Task Force to the Secretary of Health, Education and Welfare. Cambridge, MA: MIT Press, 1973.

2

Beliefs about Drugs,
Treatment, and Health

INTRODUCTION

Both a patient's and doctor's beliefs tangibly affect the patient's health. As discussed later, patients' beliefs may be shaped by their family, culture and church. A patient's belief in the value of a drug is typically called the placebo effect. Conversely, a patient's fear that a drug may cause harmful effects or that surgery will not be successful, and might result in death, is called the nocebo effect. We can also worsen our bodily symptoms based on our circumstances, our belief about what causes our symptoms, how much attention we pay to them, and our mood (Barsky, 1988, p. 22).

Cultural notions also affect our beliefs about illnesses. Some of these beliefs may even result in illnesses (called folk illnesses) that are not recognized by Western medicine (see Fishman, Bobo, Kosub, et al., 1993; Pachter, 1994). Some of these folk illnesses are discussed in the highlight box, "Other Folk Illnesses." Some folk illnesses, such as the evil eye, fulfill our need to explain why misfortune has visited our doorstep and often to place "blame" on another for our suffering (see the highlight box, "Folk Illness: The Case of the Evil Eye").

As already noted, beliefs that affect our health are influenced by cultural institutions from the family to the church. For example, in China, herbal prescriptions for various medical conditions have been handed down within families for generations (Harwood, 1981, p. 153). In this country, African Americans with diabetes are often told by black clergy that "worriation" is the cause of their increased blood sugar level (ibid., p. 76) or that faith alone, without medical treatment, can cure disease (see the interview with Levorn McCain-Jones at the end of chapter 7).

OTHER FOLK ILLNESSES

In the United States, there are beliefs about many other types of folk illnesses, including high blood (African Americans), empacho (described by various Latino ethnic groups), and geophagia (a practice common to parts of Africa and the southern United States).

High Blood

The folk illness "high blood" is not to be confused with high blood pressure. High blood is believed to result in the increased volume in the circulatory system that occurs with eating rich foods, such as red meat (Helman, 1990, p. 28). Low blood is believed to result from eating acidic foods (ibid.).

Empacho

As noted, empacho is described by many Latino ethnic groups, including Puerto Ricans, Mexicans, Mexican Americans, and Central Americans (Pachter, 1994, p. 691). It is described as food or matter that gets stuck in the walls of the stomach or intestines and then causes an obstruction. It is believed to be caused by "dietary indiscretion"— eating too much food, or food that is spoiled, eaten at the wrong time, or eaten in inappropriate combinations. It is believed to cause nausea, stomach cramps, lack of appetite, bloated stomach, or diarrhea. It is treated by dietary restrictions, herbal teas, or massage with warm oil.

Geophagia

Geophagia is the practice of eating earth or clay and is common in parts of Africa and the southern United States (ibid.). In the United States, the practice seems confined to pregnant African American women and children (ibid.). It is dangerous because it can cause gastrointestinal impaction, decreased iron absorption, and anemia (ibid.).

The belief of doctors in the value of a drug also influences patients' responses to the drug. Soon after prescription drugs are released, doctors typically have great confidence in them. This increased confidence is also conveyed to patients and is documented with enhanced health (see Benson with Stark, 1996, pp. 27–34; Frank, 1991). In fact, there is a direct correlation between the physician's enthusiasm about a therapy and its success rate (Benson with Stark, 1996, p. 34). Although it is critical to understand the role of patients' and doctors' beliefs in enhancing patients' responses to treatment, it is also important to recognize that some treatments or drugs may not fulfill the beliefs or expectations about them (see Dossey, 1993, p. 137).

Doctors' beliefs and prejudices may also negatively impact their relationship with certain patients. As discussed later, some typical prejudices within the medical establishment include those based on the social class, age, race, sex and sexual orientation of the patient.

DEVELOPING AN AWARENESS OF OUR ABILITY TO CHANGE OUR BELIEF SYSTEM

Our belief system frequently holds us back: when we believe we are not capable of certain tasks, we often fail to realize our dreams and goals; when we believe we are ugly or unworthy of having certain relationships, we give up and fail to pursue them. If we think that something is wrong with us or that we are unlovable, we probably will have "corresponding feelings associated with such beliefs—sadness, isolation and impotence" (Kaufman, 1991, p. 49). The development of such feelings is often associated with adverse health consequences.

We may not use our belief system for positive personal growth because we are not fully aware of our power to change this belief system. But we can change our belief system in an instant.[1] What is required is a decision to change (ibid., p. 109). In *Happiness Is a Choice*, Barry Kaufman shows us how people can change their belief systems in order to support themselves and their children better. Kaufman notes that parents who learn to accept the limitations of their disabled and "special needs" children will come to love them as they are, rather than expect them to "conform to our world" (ibid., p. 16). As a result, they will be more willing to engage the child in their world. For example, for the child with autism who spins plates on the floor and emits high-pitched warbling screeches, parents should not merely imitate him but "join him fully, with great sincerity and enthusiasm" (ibid.).[2]

If Viktor Frankl has taught us anything, it is that we have the capacity to view our circumstances differently. Just as those who marshaled their sense of humor even in concentration camps, we too can learn to view our circumstances more positively.

Change in our belief systems is not only critical for patients but often for doctors. Doctors who view conditions as hopeless and incurable will act accordingly (ibid., p. 110). When we speak of doctors' giving patients hope, we do not exclusively view hope as giving patients a glimpse of having a longer life but rather of allowing them to think about improving their quality of life. We must remember that there are many versions of hope, such as hope for developing peace of mind (including reducing the stress in our lives) and hope for enhancing our relationships (see the further discussion of hope in chapter 6).

FOLK ILLNESS: THE CASE OF THE EVIL EYE

The concept of the evil eye as a cause of illness is common to many cultures throughout the world, including those in the Mediterranean (Greece, Italy, Israel) and Asia (Philippines, India), Hispanic cultures (Mexico, Guatemala), and Islamic cultures (Iran, Tunisia, and Morocco) (Helman, 1990, p. 108; Maloney, 1976). In some cultures, the concept of the evil eye is similar to the concept of the evil (Sri Lanka) or hot mouth (Philippines) (Maloney, 1976, pp. 132, 149), which is believed to "cast ill through speech" (ibid., p. 151).

It is difficult to trace the origin of the evil eye, although historically, the ancient Egyptians considered the eye the seat of the soul; they also believed it had the capacity to reflect both good and evil (ibid., pp. 2–3). In modern times, however, many qualities are believed to be transmitted through the eye: in South Asia these include envy, love, wisdom, and protection (ibid., p. 130).

Jealousy and envy are believed to be main causes of the evil eye (ibid., p. 44) (newly engaged couples must be "careful" because in the village may reside envious barren women). Consequently, some measures to avoid the evil eye include: feeling reluctant to boast about one's health or express any form of admiration (ibid., pp. 65, 80, 121, 130); remaining secluded in one's home (ibid., p. 64); uttering pious phrases, particularly when admiring children (ibid., pp. 64–65); dressing in simple clothing so as not to attract attention (ibid., p. 64); or wearing amulets, ribbons, or garlic under one's clothing (ibid., p. 8).

A reluctance to compliment others is common to most peasant societies (ibid., p. 135). Reasons for this practice include the belief that praising children will spoil them (ibid.) and that individuals must be socialized to do their duty "without expecting special recognition" (ibid., p. 136).

People who cast the evil eye are believed to include those who have a physical deformity (e.g., hunchback) (ibid., p. 37); who are charismatic and successful (ibid., p. 29) (priests and popes are not immune from casting an evil eye) (ibid., p. 10); who are deviant and nonconformists (ibid., p. 64); and who are unusually thin (ibid., pp. 10, 88).

The evil eye can cause death (particularly of children), spontaneous abortion (that is why pregnant women must be cautious of those who may possess the evil eye), mental illness, and lesser symptoms, such as depression, exhaustion, and sleepiness (ibid., p. 17).

Each culture may have additional folklore surrounding the concept of the evil eye. For instance, in Italy various rituals are used to outwit "the fascination," as the evil eye is sometimes called (ibid., p. 21). A few of these rituals surround newlywed couples. One is to place a broom outside the couple's bedroom; it is said that the fascination "will be forced to count all the straws in the broom and become so tired he will lose enthusiasm for his work" (ibid.). Another is to litter the bride's bed with scraps of newspaper; since the fascination is believed to be semiliterate, it will lose time and energy reading all the scraps of paper (ibid.). In South Asia, homes are protected from the influence of the evil eye by placing a manikin of wood or one stuffed with straw and setting it upon a scaffold (ibid., p. 114). To make sure that this manikin is "irresistible," its penis is made very large and painted red (ibid.). Throughout much of the world, the colors red (Italy, South Asia) and blue (Sicily) are believed to deter the evil eye (ibid., p. 8).

The evil eye is said to be the source of economic and social control (ibid., pp. 68, 70). For example, in Tunisia, most weavers adhere to a daily production quota for the amount of cloth woven. It is reasoned that because such weavers believe in the existence of the evil eye, they adhere to these output norms so that they will not be the object of envy or jealousy. Conversely, weavers who seek to outpace the production quotas often say they need to work at home to avoid the evil eye; these weavers, however, are socially ostracized and are referred to as "ill-willed" or "antisocial" (ibid.).

In many societies, existence of the evil eye enables people to explain misfortune by providing a concrete reason for it (ibid., p. 138). By attributing misfortune to some "exterior cause," people do not have to assume personal responsibility for their illnesses (or for destruction of their crops or other property). And someone is considered the scapegoat—even though this "culpable" person is not personally implicated (ibid., p. 139).

PATIENT BELIEFS ABOUT TREATMENT

The Placebo Effect

There is strong evidence that drugs often work because patients believe that they will cause specific benefits (see Beecher, 1955). Placebos have been associated with a 30 percent success rate (Benson with Stark, 1996, p. 28), meaning that up to one third of drugs prescribed by physicians may depend upon their placebo effect (Ross & Olson, 1981). In one study, 30 percent of individuals with cancer, told they were receiving chemotherapy but actually given a placebo, experienced hair loss (Fielding, Fagg, Jones, et al., 1983). These research subjects lost their hair because they believed that chemotherapy would cause them to lose their hair! The placebo effect is enhanced when patients have heightened expectations of a drug (Benson with Stark, 1996, p. 31). In such instances, placebos have been observed to work 70–90 percent of the time (ibid., p. 30; see also Roberts, Kewman, Mercier, et al., 1993).

When used to treat pain, placebos are more likely to be effective the more intense the pain (Dossey, 1991, p. 206). The placebo effect may last for six months to one year (Benson with Stark, 1996, p. 34). Some individuals may become addicted to placebos and have withdrawal symptoms when they cease taking them (Barsky, 1988, p. 40). The placebo effect has also been reported for certain surgeries—patients' conditions improved even though the specific surgery contemplated was not performed (see Benson & McCallie, 1979; Diamond, Kittle, & Crockett, 1958).

The placebo effect varies in persons with different ethnicities (Helman, 1990, p. 172) and personalities (ibid., p. 174). Those likely to show a placebo effect have been described as being anxious, emotionally dependent, and immature, and having poor personal relationships and low self-esteem (ibid.).

The Nocebo Effect

Conversely, patients can also experience a nocebo effect and expect to become worse as a result of drug, surgical, or other treatment (see Voelker, 1996; Wade, 1996). The following scenarios and studies illustrate the nocebo effect:

- One poor and uneducated woman was seen at an emergency room with advanced breast cancer, which was "ulcerated, as large as a grapefruit and had spread to the lymph nodes in the armpit, neck and elsewhere" (Dossey, 1993, p. 123). The woman reported that this lump was visible for 15 years[3] and that she did not tell a physician about it because she believed her doctor would "cut it" and this would expose the cancer to air and make it "run wild." As a result, the woman believed she would die. Ironically, the woman finally consented to breast surgery and died shortly thereafter (ibid.).[4]
- Apparently five patients who were convinced that they would die while on the operating table did in fact die during surgery (Hackett & Weisman, 1961).

Expectations Patients Have about Particular Drugs or Treatments

Patients' expectations about a particular drug or treatment will often determine their responses to that drug or treatment. For example, varied responses to marijuana and alcohol have been attributed to the patient's belief about the nature of that response (Pihl, Segal, & Yankofsky, 1980). Marijuana may be used as a stimulant or a sleep aid (Justice, 1987, p. 297). For some it may be an aphrodisiac, whereas for others it decreases interest in sex (ibid.).

Because physiologic responses to drugs and treatments can be manipulated by conditioning, the body may be tricked into particular responses (see Ferguson, 1980, p. 254; Ikemi & Nakagawa, 1962). Consider these situations in which physiologic changes were induced by "conditioning":

- Thirteen Japanese high school students allergic to certain plants were told to close their eyes and they would be touched with a "poisonous" plant. All 13 had a reaction (from redness to blisters) even though they were not touched with a poisonous plant. Conversely, when the procedure was reversed and the boys were touched with the poisonous plant but told that it was not poisonous, only two boys had a skin reaction (Ikemi & Nakagawa, 1962).
- The immune system of a young patient with systemic lupus erythematosus was conditioned to respond to cod liver oil as if it were a powerful drug (Olness & Ader, 1992).

The immune system's ability to remember information is critical to such types of conditioning (see Ferguson, 1980, p. 254). In animal studies, if an innocent drug, one the body has not been exposed to before, is paired with an immunosuppressive one, the body will suppress its immune system when only the innocent drug is given months later (ibid.).

Beliefs about Research Protocols

Patients enrolled in research studies apparently get better faster and have better results than other patients (Benson with Stark, 1996, p. 52). This phenomenon, called the *Hawthorne effect*, is believed to be due to the fact that doctors conducting these studies may pay more attention to patients and may enthusiastically anticipate the study's results (ibid.).

Patient Compliance with Treatment

In the United Kingdom, it has been estimated that 30 percent of patients do not comply with prescribed treatment (Stimson, 1974). Patients with chronic conditions often fail to comply with therapy (Condor, 1997 [patients with AIDS]; Reichgott & Simons-Mortons, 1983 [patients with hypertension]). And at least 50 percent of patients do not take prescribed drugs correctly (Haynes, Taylor & Sackett, 1981).

Dr. Chris Costas (see interview at the end of this chapter) suggests that one reason for the long-term survival of an AIDS patient was the patient's close adherence to his treatment regimen. Some research supports this opinion. In one study, men who failed to adhere to a treatment regimen, even if it included an inert placebo, were 2.6 times more likely to die within a year than those who adhered to their medical treatment plan (Horwitz, Viscoli, Berkman, et al., 1990).

It is believed that patients do not comply with their treatment regimens for some of the following reasons:

- Once patients begin to feel well they may believe they no longer need their medication (Condor, 1997).
- Taking medications reminds patients that they are sick and different from others (Tracy, 1997). Patients with cystic fibrosis often reported a need to escape feeling different from others and this included totally neglecting their disease, not following their medication regimens, and not adhering to their need for rest (ibid.).
- Patients have known someone who eventually died despite similar drug treatment (ibid.).
- The more pills one takes per day on a complex schedule, the less likely the patient is to take all the doses ("FDA Approves 'Combivir'—Reduces Pill Regimens," 1997).
- Patients face stress (Goldston, Kovacs, Obrosky, et al., 1995). Youths with diabetes, for example, were noncompliant with treatment when they experienced various forms of life stress (ibid.).

It is believed that when a treatment plan makes sense to patients and is compatible with their life-styles, the likelihood is greater that they will comply with treatment (Roter & Hall, 1993, p. 13).

HOW PATIENTS AMPLIFY THEIR SYMPTOMS

As mentioned in the introduction, we can amplify our symptoms by the circumstances in which we find ourselves, our belief about what causes the symptoms, the amount of attention we pay to them, and our mood. Instances follow in which circumstance modulates our symptoms:

- A backache may seem worse when individuals are faced with a day of household chores as compared to engaging in pleasurable hobbies as gardening and fishing (see ibid., p. 25).
- Descriptions of the phenomenon of battlefield anesthesia have documented that soldiers in battle can disregard or be oblivious to severe wounds (Barsky, 1988, p. 24).

What we expect to feel powerfully influences what we actually feel (ibid.). As we have seen, some people who smoke marijuana expect to feel tired and others expect to feel stimulated (see Justice, 1987, p. 297). Being given a "diagnosis" may put some patients into a state of fear and panic, though others may be relieved because they now know what they have to deal with. For those for whom a diagnosis initiates panic, doctors can take concrete steps to reassure and calm them by remaining realistic yet hopeful (see chapter 6).

The context or environment in which drugs are administered also affects patient responses to them. For example, greater intoxication from marijuana occurs when it is smoked among friends than among strangers (Pihl, Segal, & Yankofsky, 1980). Tolerance to heroin is also affected by the environment in which it is used or given (Wray, 1982). The same dose of heroin that is tolerated when one uses it in familiar surroundings may be lethal when taken in unfamiliar surroundings (ibid.; see also Dossey, 1991, pp. 166–67).

If we are told, or if we believe, that we are sick, we will often behave as if we are sick. This power of suggestion was illustrated in a football stadium after some people became ill with symptoms of food poisoning. Since all the people who had become ill had consumed soft drinks, an announcement on the loudspeaker urged the fans not to patronize the dispensing machine. When this announcement was made, the entire stadium "became a sea of retching and fainting people" (Cousins, 1989, p. 82). However, with news that the dispensing machine was not a cause of the illness, symptoms vanished as suddenly as they had appeared (ibid.). Our capacity to follow the path of our expectations explains, as discussed later, the increased mortality rate of persons who are well but believe they are sick.

People who have serious diseases (or who believe they have a serious disease) often perceive all future symptoms as evidence of disease progression. In a study of patients who had a chest x-ray and were told that further testing was needed because of possible abnormality, one tenth experienced new or increased symptoms that they thought were caused by heart disease (Wheeler, Williamson, & Cohen, 1958).

Concentrating on one's body increases the number of symptoms that will be reported, and concentrating on a particular bodily sensation intensifies it (Pennebaker, 1982). People who report many bodily symptoms also report many psychological symptoms, such as feeling moody or being more high strung or easily hurt (ibid., pp. 135–39; see Mechanic, 1979).

Patient Beliefs about Their Health

Patients' assessments of their health are closely associated with mortality (see Idler, 1992; Schoenfeld, Malmrose, Blazer, et al., 1994). People who are healthy but who believe they are sick often have an increased risk of death. For example, those who say their health is poor are seven times more likely to die than those who say their health is excellent (Dossey, 1991, p. 16).

Patients and physicians often view the patient's health in quite different ways. Patients are two to three times more likely to rate their health as better than their physicians do (Roter & Hall, 1993, p. 8). When patients' prognoses are unknown, patients may believe that they have a chance of healing or survival (see Dossey, 1993, p. 123).

HOW DOCTORS' BELIEFS MAY PROMOTE
OR THREATEN SURVIVAL

Doctors can have extraordinary effects on their patients—their words, attitudes, and beliefs can support or destroy the trust in the doctor/patient relationship. A doctor's words can determine whether the patient feels hope or despair. A doctor's beliefs may influence the patient's response to treatment. For example, when doctors thought they were giving patients morphine, the placebo was twice as effective as when they thought they were administering a mild analgesic (Frank, 1991). The mere presence of the doctor, an authority figure, evokes particular responses in patients, including elevated blood pressure (Lynch, 1983, p. 185).

HOW PREJUDICES IN HEALTH AND MEDICINE
AFFECT TREATMENT OF PATIENTS

The medical establishment, including doctors, often treats different groups of patients differently. Such discrimination may sometimes be subtle and unintended; in other instances it may be quite overt and calculated. This discrimination can be based on such factors as social class and ability to pay (based on insurance status), race and ethnicity, age, gender, and sexual orientation.

Discrimination Based on Socioeconomic Status and Insurance Status

Discrimination based on patients' abilities to pay, related to their social class and whether they have insurance, is well documented (Burstin, Lipsitz, & Brennan, 1992; Sorlie, Johnson, Backlund, et al., 1994). Several investigators, however, have tried to determine how socioeconomic and insurance status affect health outcomes for patients and whether these variables are independent of each other. Burstin, Lipsitz, and Brennan have reported that the uninsured have a *twofold* greater risk of being injured through negligent care than those with insurance, even when controlling for race, gender, and income (Burstin, Lipsitz, & Brennan, 1992). Sorlie, Johnson, Backlund, et al., however, have reported that for patients within each health insurance group (i.e., patients on Medicaid, on Medicare, or without insurance), mortality rate unequivocally decreases with increasing income (Sorlie, Johnson, Backlund, et al., 1994). This latter study, therefore, indicates that one's socioeconomic status is a greater predictor of mortality, independent of health insurance status (ibid.).

Uninsured or underinsured patients are often transferred from hospitals with a large percentage of insured patients to public hospitals (Schiff, Ansell, Schlosser, et al., 1986). This practice, called "patient dumping," is particularly shocking because patients are often transferred when their medical condition is unstable. Consequently, one study reported that 39 percent of the unstable patients transferred to a public hospital were admitted to its intensive care unit (Schiff, Ansell, Schlosser, et al. 1986, p. 554) and over 9 percent of such patients who were transferred died (ibid.).

Uninsured patients *may* receive medical care that is inferior to that given to those with insurance. Patients with lung cancer who were uninsured were less likely than insured patients to undergo surgery, chemotherapy, and radiation (Greenberg, Chute, Stukel, et al., 1988)—arguably "medically necessary" treatments for cancer.

Uninsured patients also often have fewer procedures done than patients with some form of insurance. For example, researchers who examined over 37,000 hospital records of patients treated for cardiovascular problems, who had private insurance, no insurance, or Medicaid, found that payer status was strongly associated with use of expensive cardiac procedures (Wenneker, Weissman, & Epstein, 1990). Others have noted, however, that groups of patients who undergo fewer procedures may not necessarily be discriminated against—they argue that patients who undergo more procedures may be overtreated (Hadley, Steinberg, & Feder, 1991). And some have distinguished between "medically necessary" and discretionary procedures, arguing that payer status affects the use of discretionary but not medically necessary care (ibid.).

Discrimination Based on Race

In the United States, racism in the medical establishment can be illustrated by the Tuskegee syphilis experiment, in which the government purposefully exposed black men to syphilis in order to study the natural course of the disease (see Jones, 1981). Although an effective treatment was developed for syphilis by the middle of the study, these men were never told about it and never treated (ibid.). This and other types of discrimination still form the basis of much mistrust of the American medical establishment among African Americans. In light of this distrust, it is not surprising that only 12 percent of African American men with human immunodeficiency virus/acquired immunodeficiency syndrome (HIV/AIDS) in one study took protease inhibitors (compared with 33 percent of white patients) (Whitfield, 1997).

More subtle forms of racism by the American health and medical establishments certainly include receipt of fewer medical services and less effort to educate and target African Americans with preventive medicine. In the United States, African Americans receive fewer recommendations for open heart surgery despite equal clinical need (Maynard, Fisher, & Passamani, 1986).

Much racial discrimination has been documented by mental health professionals. The stereotype, for example, that blacks are violent has often been the basis for their disparate treatment. Consider the following information:

- One study considered the pattern of referrals in a small Massachusetts town and found that blacks were overwhelmingly sent to a local correctional facility, while their white counterparts who exhibited the same level of psychopathological and violent behavior tended to be referred to local mental health hospitals (Lewis, Shanok, Cohen, et al., 1980).

- In a psychiatric setting, black youth were four times more likely than whites to be physically restrained for similar acts of aggression (Bond, DiCandia, & MacKinnon, 1988).

- Black psychiatric patients with case information closely related to that of white patients are often given a more severe diagnosis because they are stereotyped as more dangerous (Loring & Powell, 1988). In the United States, black psychiatric patients are more likely be diagnosed as "schizophrenic" (Strakowski, Lonczak, Sax, et al., 1995). In the United Kingdom, racial prejudice is also illustrated by the fact that Afro-Caribbean patients are classified by psychiatrists as mad even when there is evidence to the contrary (Helman, 1990, p. 65).

Apart from the existence of racial discrimination, the *effects* of racial discrimination are often quite profound. Several studies have documented the relationship between elevated blood pressure and the experience of racial discrimination (Krieger & Sidney, 1996). And in the mental health context, the consequence of being diagnosed with a psychotic disorder means that one is less likely to have outpatient treatment or be treated by a professional therapist (Flaskerud & Hu, 1992).

Black patients are also overrepresented in involuntary hospitalizations in public mental hospitals, and, as a result, they are also less likely to be referred to community-based programs (Wade, 1993). When patients are involuntarily admitted to mental hospitals, they are more significantly deprived of their civil liberties than when they are treated in outpatient settings. In *Vitek v. Jones*, the Supreme Court recognized that with an involuntary admission to such a hospital, patients not only lose their liberty, because they are confined against their will, but they face the added stigma of being characterized as "mentally ill." Conversely, when patients are treated in outpatient settings, they are usually free to accept or decline treatment and their freedom to go from place to place is not restricted.

Discrimination Based on Age

Physicians raise and discuss fewer psychosocial issues with the elderly than with younger patients who have similar issues (Roter & Hall, 1993, p. 41). Some physicians are suggesting that as our population ages doctors will need to be more aware of the close relationship between psychological issues facing the elderly and their health, as illustrated by the following scenario:

An elderly man was seen with pneumonia but because his condition responded to treatment the interns and residents found it "uninteresting." Apparently, the man's grief at the loss of his wife caused him to become depressed and this depression became associated with a loss of appetite. Furthermore, the man's swollen knee made it difficult for him to go up and down stairs and, consequently, he didn't go out for groceries.

Because malnourishment (and most likely depression) weakened his immune system, he was more susceptible to a bacterial infection. One night he started to drink and became intoxicated. He vomited and aspirated some vomitus into his lungs. Within two weeks, he came back to the emergency room with aspiration pneumonia. (Longino, 1997)

Related to discrimination based on age is the lack of public policy to address the needs of our aging population. Ironically, this public policy will likely be framed by the younger among us.[5] Those within academic medicine recognize that many physicians will be needed in the next 40 years to care for the elderly (Caelleigh, 1997). In 2030 it is projected that over 70 million people in the United States will be over 65 years of age (ibid.). Before appropriate public and medical policy can be adopted to meet the needs of the elderly, several critical factors should be considered:

- The lack of knowledge about the stages of development for those 60 years and older—some have suggested that "virtually nothing" is known about such stages of development (ibid.).
- The failure of doctors to apply "their science and skills to the one sure part of medicine, the death of patients" probably because they "have too often turned away from patients [that] cannot [be] cure[d]" (ibid.).
- The fact that the elderly may need systems that are "high touch" and "low tech" (ibid.).

Sexism and Discrimination Based on Gender

Historically, the medical establishment has been rife with sexism and gender-based discrimination (Marieskind, 1980; Ruzek, 1978; Weisman, 1998). Such sexism and discrimination has occurred through

- the overuse of surgery on women (e.g., hysterectomies and sterilizations);
- the use of particularly risky drugs and devices (e.g., diethylstilbestrol [DES] and intrauterine devices) in women's bodies;
- the medicalization of women's reproductive functions (e.g., the birthing process and artificial insemination);
- the condescending manner in which women have been treated by health professionals, including doctors and mental health professionals.

Hysterectomies and sterilizations have been overused on women; a study by the Columbia School of Public Health found that one third of 6,248 hysterectomies reviewed were without medical justification (Ruzek, 1978, p. 49, citing The Boston Women's Health Book Collective, *Our Bodies, Ourselves,* 1973). Some believe that the abuse of women's bodies with unnecessary hysterectomies occurred merely to "collect a fee."[6] As women enter the surgical specialties, it is unclear whether they will perform fewer hysterectomies than men (Bickell, Earp, Garrett, et al., 1994 [men will perform more hysterectomies]; Geller, Burns, & Brailler, 1996 [women will perform fewer hysterectomies]).

The record of involuntary sterilization is another shocking example of sexism and gender-based discrimination against women. In 1942, the United States Supreme Court declared the Oklahoma Habitual Criminal Sterilization Act unconstitutional (*Skinner v. Oklahoma*). This act, which ordered the sterilization of anyone convicted of three crimes involving "moral turpitude," was found to violate the "right to procreate," and, therefore, the Court said, this right could only be abridged for a "compelling state interest." Beginning in the 1950s, many states repealed legislation permitting eugenic sterilization "for institutionalized persons or limited the powers of conservators and guardians to 'procure' sterilization" (Reich, 1995, p. 844). But in 1973 two sterilization cases received national prominence—they were obtained without informed consent of the patients or their guardians and involved obvious coercion by the doctors involved. In the first case, two black girls ages 12 and 14 were sterilized in a federally funded family planning clinic[7] in Alabama (Ruzek, 1978, p. 47). Their informed consent was not obtained and their mother was "persuaded" to give her consent by signing an X on a form she could not read (ibid.); the mother was also not told that the procedure was "permanent" (ibid.). The second case involved a South Carolina obstetrician who refused to deliver a third child to a welfare mother unless she consented to sterilization (ibid.). Ruzek believes that since 1970 sterilizations have "increased rapidly" (ibid.), although involuntary sterilizations such as those involving coercion have probably been confined to minorities (Kelly, 1997 [Native Americans]; Ruzek, 1978, p. 47).

The medical establishment's use of risky drugs and devices in women's bodies has also historically illustrated its sexism—in complicity with pharmaceutical companies and federal regulatory agencies such as the Food and Drug Administration. DES, which was prescribed as an agent to prevent spontaneous abortion—despite some medical evidence to the contrary[8]—is just one example of a drug that was later identified to produce vaginal cancer in the children of mothers who used the drug (Ruzek, 1978, pp. 38–39). The intrauterine devices (IUDs) are just one product implanted in a woman's body and subsequently found to be unsafe (ibid., pp. 43–46). IUDs have been documented to cause miscarriage and in some situations death (e.g., by 1974, 36 women in the United States had died because they had used an IUD) (ibid., p. 43).

The medicalization of women's reproductive functions is another instance of sexism in the medical establishment—evidence of how a male-oriented profession has sought to make decisions for women that might best be left to them. Historically, birthing has been a glaring example of the medicalization of women's reproductive functions (ibid., p. 17). In the early 1900s male doctors waged "war" on midwives and succeeded in outlawing midwifery in spite of opinions such as those of a Johns Hopkins physician who in 1912 expressed his belief that most American doctors were less competent than midwives because they were unreliable at preventing uterine infections and neonatal blindness (ibid.).

Artificial insemination (AI) is yet another service that has been "medicalized" (Weisman, 1998, p. 22). However, at women's health centers, women are increasingly performing AI on themselves using turkey basters and a donor's semen (Wikler & Wikler, 1991): in essence, attempting to demedicalize this procedure. Demedicalization particularly benefits lesbians, who, for reasons discussed later, often are refused AI services by physicians and other health professionals. However, the law clearly favors medicalization of AI and often imposes harsh penalties on women who must seek the services of persons other than physicians in order to obtain the procedure. Three states impose a penalty for non-physician-assisted AI—and Georgia makes it a felony (ibid., p. 22). Additionally, many states hold that the sperm donor will have rights and responsibilities of fatherhood only if the insemination is supervised by a physician (ibid., p. 21). And there has already been a California case in which a court awarded visitation to the sperm donor because the insemination was arranged nonmedically (*Jhordan C. v. Mary K.*, 1986).

Last, the condescending way in which women have been treated by health professionals is further evidence of medical sexism. This condescension can take many forms, such as the following:

- Treating a woman as if she were incapable of making a decision—and many have suggested that male doctors treat women as if they are children (Broverman, Broverman, Clarkson, et al., 1970; Roth & Lerner, 1974)—such that it is difficult "for women to acquire information they need to make competent decisions" (Ruzek, 1978, p. 34).
- Treating a woman as if her husband mattered more than she (Scully & Bart, 1973): In an analysis of 27 of the 32 general gynecology texts published in the United States since 1943, Scully and Bart noted that women were consistently described as "anatomically destined to reproduce, nurture and *keep their husbands happy*" (emphasis added) (ibid.).
- Failing to respect the patient: For example, in a study on racism and health care, pregnant African American women were considered to receive care that was "indifferent, inaccessible, and undignified" (Murrell, Smith, Gill, et al., 1996).
- Failing to credit a woman's symptoms, such as viewing a woman as a complainer— and 72 percent of doctors when asked to describe a typical complaining patient have spontaneously described a woman (Cooperstock, 1971). Some women believe that as they age, male physicians "talk down" to them and do not fully credit the alleged extent of their symptoms (see the interview with Charlotte Streit). This has caused Charlotte Streit to avoid treatment by male physicians.

Discrimination Based on Sexual Orientation

Several polls have indicated that physicians are prejudiced against gays and lesbians. In a survey of general practitioners, only 32.7 percent reported feeling comfortable with gay men (Bhugra, 1989). In a survey of the psychiatric faculty of a medical school, 25 percent admitted to being prejudiced against homosexuals (Chaimowitz, 1991). More recent polls of first- and second-year medical students, however, show a shift in opinion: 80 percent of students who had gay and lesbian acquaintances had a high level of knowledge about homosexuality ("Health and Science," 1998).

It may be questionable what physicians actually know about homosexuality since apparently only three and one half hours is devoted to the topic during the four-year medical curriculum (Wallick, Cambre, & Townsend, 1992). Many gays and lesbians do not disclose their sexual orientation to their doctors, fearing their doctors will despise them. Apparently only one third of lesbians disclose their sexual orientation to their doctors (*Searching for Women*, 1992, p. 52). According to a poll in *The Advocate*, a leading American gay and lesbian magazine, 55 percent of female and male respondents reported having had "difficulty" discussing their sexuality with their gynecologist or primary care physician. In a study of 632 English homosexual men, 44 percent had never informed their general practitioners of their sexual orientation (Fitzpatrick, Dawson, Boulton, et al., 1994). Some studies have even reported that gay men with HIV/AIDS do not disclose their HIV status to their physicians. Of 77 English homosexuals who were HIV-positive, 44 percent had not told their doctors their diagnosis (ibid.).

There are tangible health consequences when gays and lesbians fail to talk honestly about their sexual orientation with their physicians. Consider the following examples:

- For lesbians, many issues might be ignored simply because they are not heterosexual (see "The Advocate Poll," 1997). Other issues, however, such as artificial insemination, though relevant to lesbians, are often considered too controversial by the medical establishment[9] (largely because of the belief of the importance of the father in child rearing[10] and the idea that the mother's lesbian identity will influence the child's gender development).[11] In addition to the medical aspects of AI, there are substantial legal problems that may arise if the couple is not a married heterosexual couple.[12]

- Gay men are at greater risk for hepatitis B and anal cancer than heterosexual men ("Health Care Needs of Gay Men and Lesbians in the United States," 1996). In fact, gay men's risk for anal cancer is 25–84 times higher than that of heterosexuals (ibid.).

- The prevalence of substance abuse among homosexuals ranges from 28 to 35 percent compared to 10 to 12 percent for heterosexuals ("Patients Don't Always Reveal Their Sexual Orientation," 1996).

- For gay (and bisexual) male adolescents, the risk of suicide is substantial. Data from various North American studies indicate that the lifetime attempted suicide rate has tripled, from 9.6 percent in 1950 to 31.3 percent in 1990 for this population (see Bagley & Tremblay, 1997). This also appears to be the case in other countries.[13]

BELIEFS BASED ON THE PATIENT'S FAMILY, COMMUNITY, RACE, OR ETHNICITY

Beliefs Particular to Families

Beliefs that we may have acquired, on the basis of how we were treated by our families, are believed to influence health. Certain personality traits in those with psychosomatic disorders often developed as a reaction to treatment in one's family of origin (Minuchin, Rosman, & Baker, 1978). In China, families hand down prescriptions for herbal remedies from generation to generation (Harwood, 1981, p. 153), and this custom may affect the health of their descendants.

Beliefs Particular to Certain Cultures and Communities

In some cultures, being sick is practically romanticized (see Ohnuki-Tierney, 1989, p. 62); in others being sick is believed to be the result of one's moral conduct: this view is related to the concept that the sick are somehow morally reprehensible or "contaminated" (see Appiah-Kubi, 1989, p. 213). For example, the Japanese are "fond" of illnesses and view someone who is completely healthy as "unintelligent or lacking some desirable quality" (Ohnuki-Tierney, 1989, p. 62).[14] In the 1820s, those with tuberculosis (TB) were considered genteel and even creative (Sontag, 1978, p. 28); because of this, the disappearance of TB was associated with the decline of literature and the arts (ibid., p. 32).

But some cultures view the sick as morally polluted (this topic is extensively discussed in chapter 3). For example, the Akan of Ghana view health and disease as "inextricably connected with socially approved behavior and moral conduct" (Appiah-Kubi, 1989, p. 213).

There is not much information on how the values and moral perspectives of the communities in which patients live influence their health-related decisions (see Carrese & Rhodes, 1995). Doctors must understand how patients' communities affect their health-related beliefs and how these communities may become patients' source of strength, help them achieve a sense of self-worth and identity, and even make decisions for them. For instance, Mexican American families often participate in what amounts to making a joint decision with the patient (Harwood, 1981, p. 316).

Beliefs Based on Race or Ethnicity

Beliefs about Receiving Bad News. For traditional Navahos, discussing the occurrence of symptoms or of medical "bad news," like the possibility of illness, is believed to result in the occurrence of such illness/symptoms (ibid.). Many

Asians believe that discussing cancer or other diseases may cause their occurrence (Aoki, Ngin, Mo, et al., 1989, p. 296).

As a result of these beliefs, doctors find it difficult to discuss the risks of surgery with Navaho patients. One Navaho woman, speaking of how the risks of bypass surgery were communicated to her father, noted that "[t]he surgeon told him that he may not wake up, that this is the risk of every surgery. For the surgeon it was very routine, but the way that my Dad received it, it was almost like a death sentence, and he never consented to the surgery" (Carrese & Rhodes, 1995).

Some have suggested that the difficulty of receiving bad news, for groups such as certain Native Americans or Asians, may make any discussion of planning for future disability (e.g., the discussion of advance directives like powers of attorney or living wills) difficult (ibid.). Advance directives conflict with the traditional Navaho belief that one should seek to live as long as possible on earth. Consequently, it is inconceivable to consider shortening this period. A study of 22 Navaho patients showed that only 14 percent considered advance directives "somewhat acceptable" (ibid.).

Beliefs about the Treatment of Disease. Many ethnic groups have strong views about the treatment of disease. Hispanics, for example, are often proponents of nontraditional forms of therapy, and, as a result, they

- share prescription medications among family members and friends (Jacobsen, 1994);
- use herbal medicine extensively (Smith, Lin, & Mendoza, 1993); and
- consult spiritists on a frequent basis: about 30–40 percent of Puerto Ricans in the general population consult spiritists (Harwood, 1981, p. 423).

CHAPTER SUMMARY

Both patients' and doctors' belief systems may profoundly affect their adaptation to living and ultimately their health. All persons should realize that they have the capacity to change their lives by changing their present experiences. They do this when they decide to change their belief systems, which, according to Barry Kaufman, can be changed in an instant and can dramatically affect our physical and psychosocial health. Such changes can help us to preserve our peace of mind even though our bodies are ravaged by disease; accept our "special needs" children such that our love enables us really to communicate with them; and view ourselves as healthy even though our bodies may be affected by physical disease. It has been noted that those who say their health is poor are seven times more likely to die than those who say their health is excellent.

Patients also have particular beliefs about either the positive or the negative effects of the medicines they may take and procedures they may undergo. These beliefs have been observed and characterized as the placebo and nocebo effects, respectively. Patients who expect that a drug will produce a given reaction will experience that reaction about 33 percent of the time even if they are given a placebo or sugar pill. The placebo effect is further enhanced when patients have heightened expectations regarding a drug, as when they are newly marketed and doctors are enthusiastic about their efficacy. Amazingly, the placebo effect can last for six months to one year. Conversely, when patients expect to be harmed by or to die from a drug or treatment, this often occurs.

Patients' beliefs are profoundly affected by their culture and even by their families and churches. In some cultures, for example, illness is romanticized, whereas in others the ill are seen as social and moral reprobates. In some cultures, illness is even believed to be influenced by diet (e.g., the belief that some conditions are caused by an imbalance of "hot" or "cold" and that certain foods can remedy this imbalance).

Doctors' beliefs also profoundly affect patients' health. It is also the case that, when doctors have thought they were giving patients morphine, the placebo effect was twice as pronounced as when they thought they were giving a mild analgesic. Doctors' beliefs also reflect their prejudices. Several studies suggest that sexism, racism, homophobia, classism, and ageism exist in the medical profession.

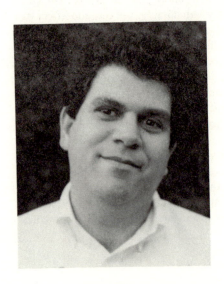

AN INTERVIEW WITH CHRIS COSTAS

I'm board-certified in pediatrics, internal medicine and infectious disease. I've been in practice since 1988 and currently work as a hospital epidemiologist in a Catholic-affiliated community-based hospital. This hospital is located in the suburbs of a large metropolitan area. At the hospital, I see patients with AIDS (mostly intravenous drug users who are uninsured), babies in a pediatric clinic (one morning per week), and patients in the hospital with severe infections. I also work in a holistic health clinic, not affiliated with the hospital I work at, where I treat patients with Chinese acupuncture and herbs.

I am interested in doctor/patient communication dynamics and am knowledgeable about the eastern and western views of such dynamics. In the Chinese system, the Yellow Emperor's textbook cautioned doctors to first attempt to heal a person with words. I have found words to work in the treatment of anger and anxiety. I also use "hakomi communication skills" when speaking to patients. With this communication style, the speaker can open with a "contact statement," which describes what the doctor believes the patient feels. I often make contact with my patients with AIDS by saying "Gee, you look sad today." Hakomi communication skills demand that you listen attentively to what the patient has said—and this accomplishes what is in fact a great desire on the part of patients—to be listened to. Other hakomi communication skills focus on what the patient may expect from you as well as trying to elicit where the patient is spiritually. In any event, questions should be open-ended and non-judgmental.

Unfortunately, some doctors are judgmental. I once saw an orthopedic surgeon for plantar fascitis (pain in my heel) which made it difficult for me to run. I used to run 40 miles per week but with the fascitis could only run five miles. When the surgeon found out how much I used to run, he said "that's too much for your age" (I was 39 years old at the time). I found this comment judgmental because I had no underlying heart or other condition that should have restricted the amount I ran. Furthermore, I used running as a vehicle for meditation, stress-reduction and prayer—outlets I'm sure the surgeon did not realize. My fascitis was ultimately cured by a practitioner of chi gong (or "Qigong")—from a Western perspective, chi gong may be considered a form of positive thinking which combines meditation, breath control, and gymnastics (Porkert with Ullmann, 1982, p. 106). Chi gong essentially induces a whole-body relaxation response (Benson with Proctor, 1984, pp. 100–101). Central to the philosophy of chi gong is "the understanding that we must cultivate moral and physical strength together to prolong life, develop human potential and help others" (Guo, 1996).

As a pediatrician, I'm familiar with the concept of treating the entire family, not just the sick child. I use this model when treating people with AIDS, although I'm aware that, in general, the medical profession often focuses on the patient and ignores the reality that the family may need to receive medical information and support. I always ask my patients with AIDS if they want me to speak to their biological or "alternative" families. I do this to ensure that the patient has a support network. Such a network makes the patient more likely to comply with medical treatment and to be less isolated (people with AIDS are still isolated but less so than when the epidemic began).

I was the doctor for one man with AIDS who lived for seven years with virtually no T-cells. I attribute this man's longevity to: his social support (he belonged to a religious cult that supported him), self-care (good nutrition and exercise); his following medical advice, and taking an active role in deciding his treatment regimen. He reviewed the medical literature and looked objectively at studies of the effectiveness of drugs used to treat HIV/AIDS.

My criticism of the medical profession is that treatment is problem-specific (meaning that in any given encounter with the patient, usually only one problem is addressed), that the system is tiered and is profit-motivated (meaning that the system completely honors the needs of patients with money), and that only traditional therapies are considered valid.

SUGGESTED READING

Beinfield, Harriet, and Efren Korngold. *Between Heaven and Earth: A Guide to Chinese Medicine.* New York: Ballantine, 1992.

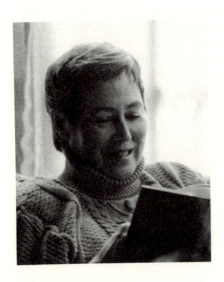

AN INTERVIEW WITH CHARLOTTE STREIT

I am 56 years old and have had osteoarthritis/fibromyalgia for 15 years and rheumatoid arthritis for three years. I also suffer from "heel spurs," a congenital back condition, and limited range of motion in my neck due to "frozen" vertebrae. After a "flare-up" two years ago of all these forms of arthritis, I chose to take the anti-cancer drug methotrexate, which was considered "experimental" for the treatment of arthritis, to relieve my pain and discomfort. Unfortunately, late in the first year, the drug caused me to develop double pneumonia and I was put in the hospital. After 10 days, I was home but I had to continue the oxygen support for the next four months. I am now using the anti-inflammatory drug Relafen.

The symptoms from arthritis, mainly constant pain, stiffness and depression, began when I neared age 40. Secondary symptoms have included increased weight gain and fatigue. I also have hypertension and high cholesterol, which I believe is worsened by the stress of dealing with arthritis.

Up until this year, I knew I should exercise and be aware of the way I was eating, but the pain was so bad that at times a good day for me was to make it down the stairs and do a little light housework. (A hard thing to take for a woman who used to run three to five miles a day!) The increased depression and frustration of what was happening to my body seemed to create a vicious cycle.

Although I have had some fine male doctors, I currently am being seen solely by women physicians. In looking back, I found that most male doctors treated me with insensitivity, were distant and, at times, intimidating. They said they were "sorry" I was tired, stiff, and in pain, but they couldn't find the cause. Some gave me the feeling that I should not be "complaining," that "a person of my age should expect a few aches and pains." I think they felt I was pre-menopausal and it was all in my head. I just started menopause a year ago!

Such responses gave me the resolve to see if I could help myself. I turned to the local library where I found many interesting books on arthritis—there are over 100 types of arthritis alone! So, I began to educate myself on the diverse nature of arthritis and ways to get around some of the limitations it imposed. It was through reading that I was finally able to have my fibromyalgia diagnosed and to learn ways to reduce its pain. I also learned about "heel spurs" and found a podiatrist who x-rayed my feet, found I had them, and recommended orthodics—these eliminated the need for surgery.

Today, I delight and take much encouragement from my women doctors. I'm finding that they seem to take a more collaborative approach, forming a partnership for healing with me. They also have the insight to ask me what, if anything, is going on in other areas of my life. Because the male doctors caused me to feel like a "complainer," I found that when I started seeing my woman rheumatologist, I was pretty guarded and reluctant to report symptoms, such as when the methotrexate affected my lungs. As I have experienced my doctor's empathy and her desire to fully understand me, I am less guarded and more willing to describe my symptoms. I also like the way women seem to take time with me and to see the arthritis through my eyes.

Over the ensuing years, as I have "fought" this disease, I have been made aware of not only the physical but also the psychological, spiritual, and mental nature of suffering. I am coming to believe that we must be keenly aware of the connection between mind, body, and spirit with regard to healing and well-being. Having had an alcoholic father, I experienced the stress it puts on the children and the way we internalize it. My mother was sick a lot and as the only girl with four brothers, I was the "feeler," the little mother on whom everyone relied, so I took on everyone's pain. By the time I was through high school, my childhood headaches had become terrible migraines. These continued to plague me until I was in my early 40s. And like many from this kind of environment, I married a man with a drinking problem. In going through the Adult Children of Alcoholics and Al-Anon programs, and with therapy, I began the journey of letting go, dealing with the pain in my life and learning to nurture and take care of myself. I finally was able to see that the family I was brought up in, the church I belonged to, and the society that conditioned me, were factors in the way I saw myself.

Although illness has sometimes robbed me of strength and tested my hope, with the help, compassion, enthusiasm, and humor of my loved ones, dear friends, kind therapists, and my own faith life, I am able to mobilize myself to fight. I don't believe I was ever afraid to suffer. My fear was that I would have to go through it alone, not knowing what my suffering was about. What a joy to know I am not in this fight alone.

I have learned to open myself to alternative treatments such as acupuncture, chi gong (or "Qigong") (for a definition of chi gong, see the prior interview with Chris Costas), massage therapy, Tai Chi, music, swimming, meditation, prayer, and stress management. I am also supplementing my medicine with vitamins and antioxidants and a few alternative medicines. I am hoping that this will allow me to reduce the amount of anti-inflammatory drugs I take. In this milieu, I have begun to find the way to increased hope, energy, understanding, weight loss, and a more peace-filled outlook for the future. I believe that partnership, trust, and cooperation is essential to working with your doctor. I realize that I should be, and I am learning to be, in charge of my own health and well-being.

SUGGESTED READINGS

On Arthritis

Fries, James F. *Arthritis: A Comprehensive Guide to Understanding Your Arthritis*, 3rd ed. Reading, MA: Addison-Wesley, 1990.
Kushner, Irving, ed. *Understanding Arthritis*. New York: Charles Scribner's Sons, 1984.
Lorig, Kate, and James F. Fries. *The Arthritis Helpbook: A Tested Self-Management Program for Coping with Your Arthritis*, 3rd ed. Reading, MA: Addison-Wesley, 1990.

On Chronic Illness

Schmidt, Stephen A. *Living with Chronic Illness: The Challenge of Adjustment*. Minneapolis, MN: Augsburg Publishing House, 1989.

Religious/Spiritual

Estes, Clarissa P. *Women Who Run with the Wolves: Myths and Stories of the Wild Women Archetype*. New York: Ballantine, 1992.
Whitehead, Evelyn E., and James D. Whitehead. *Season of Strength: New Visions of Adult Christian Maturing*. Winona, MN: St. Mary's Press, 1994.

NOTES

1. Those who spend years in psychotherapy do not change their belief systems in an instant or in a short period of time. But this does not mean that it cannot be done.

2. Barry Kaufman has also described how he and his spouse dealt with the autism of their son. He reports that after working

with him twelve hours a day, seven days a week for over three years, this mute, dysfunctioning, severely retarded, under-30 I.Q. autistic child blossomed into a highly verbal, extroverted, expressive and loving youngster, who bore absolutely no traces of his original condition. Raun went on to display a near-genius I.Q. and maintained an almost straight "A" academic average in both grade school and high school, graduating with honors. Currently, he attends one of the finest universities in the country, loves tennis, volleyball and cross-country skiing and lights up our home with his unending curiosity, wit and laughter. (Kaufman, 1991, p. 17)

3. Statistically it is considered impossible for a person to live for 15 years with untreated breast cancer, particularly after it has become visible (Dossey, 1993, p. 123).

4. The belief that one should not "cut" a cancer and expose it to air has some support in the African American community (Jackson & Nixon, 1970).

5. According to Irving Rosow, "The crucial people in the aging problem are not the old, but the younger age groups, for it is the rest of us who determine the status and position of the old person in the social order" (Rosow, 1962).

6. Seaman suggested that the abuse of hysterectomy was done merely to collect a fee. It was noted that when a plan for reimbursement of surgical fees was offered to the United Mine Workers, excessive surgical bills were submitted (Seaman, 1972, pp. 190–93). However, when the Mine Workers required preop consultations, because of increased rates for gynecological surgery, hysterectomy rates decreased by as much as 75 percent (ibid.).

7. Federal regulations now provide for special informed consent procedures and a "waiting period" for federally funded sterilizations. See "Sterilization of Persons in Federally Assisted Programs of the Public Health Service," 42 C.F.R. § 50, 201 et seq. (1993); "Sterilizations," 42 C.F.R. § 441.250 et seq. (1993).

8. Apparently the medical literature contained at least six medical articles that concluded that DES was ineffective in preventing spontaneous abortion (Ruzek, 1978, p. 39).

9. Donor insemination of lesbian couples remains controversial both in the United States and in most European fertility centers (Brewaeys, Ponjaert, Van Hall, et al., 1997). In the United States, the ethical committee of the American Society for Reproductive Medicine has stressed that "the child's best interest is served when it is born and reared in an environment of a heterosexual couple in a stable marriage" (American Society of Reproductive Medicine, 1994). In the European community, it appears that donor insemination of lesbian couples is discouraged by the belief of the importance of a father figure in a child's life (Brewaeys, Ponjaert, Van Hall, et al., 1997).

10. In a meta analysis of 67 empirical studies of the effect of a father's absence on the child's gender role development, no overall differences were found between children brought up with and without a father (Stevenson & Black, 1988; see also Kirkpatrick, 1988).

11. In the first study to trace the children of lesbian mothers from youth to adulthood, no significant difference in sexual orientation between the children of lesbian mothers

and those of heterosexual mothers was reported (Golombok & Tasker, 1996). This study was begun in 1976 and 1977 with 27 lesbian mothers and their 39 children, who were then an average age of nine and one half years. In the follow-up in 1992 and 1993, 26 daughters and 20 sons were interviewed.

12. The most widespread legislative approach has been to facilitate AI for married heterosexuals "by providing a method for them to proceed with some guarantee that they will have exclusive paternal rights" ("Reproductive Technologies," 1995, p. 2219). Lesbians and the gay men who have often been their sperm donors must wade through much murky legal territory (see Chira, 1993; Dunlap, 1994). In the case of a gay man in San Francisco who donated his sperm so that a lesbian couple could have a child, the donor was granted legal standing as the child's father (Dunlap, 1994). Yet a Boston court allowed Dr. Susan Love and Dr. Helen Cooksey to adopt a five-year-old daughter, conceived by Dr. Love with sperm donated from Dr. Cooksey's cousin (Chira, 1993) and, therefore, granted both mothers full parental rights.

13. Gays and lesbians aged 15–25 in Belgium's Flanders region are two to five times more likely to attempt suicide than straight youth ("Belgian Gay and Lesbian Youths More Likely to Attempt Suicide," 1998). Lifetime rates of suicidal behavior range from 20 to 50 percent (mean, 31.3 percent) in North America, and similar rates have been reported for community-based samples of British gay youth (Plummer, 1989).

14. Ironically, however, the Japanese stigmatize those suffering from genetic diseases such as hemophilia (Feldman & Yonemoto, 1992).

SUGGESTED READINGS

Benson, Herbert, with Marg Stark. *Timeless Healing: The Power of Biology and Belief.* New York: Scribner, 1996.

Ruzek, Sheryl Burt. *The Women's Health Movement: Feminist Alternatives to Medical Control.* New York: Praeger, 1978.

Smith, James Monroe. *AIDS and Society.* Upper Saddle River, NJ: Prentice-Hall, 1996 (chapter 3 on prejudice discusses prejudice against gays and lesbians and people with HIV/AIDS).

REFERENCES

"The Advocate Poll: Sexuality at the Doctor's Office." *The Advocate*, Oct. 28, 1997, p. 6.

American Society of Reproductive Medicine. "Ethical Guidelines for the Use of DI." 62 (Supp. 1) *Fertility & Sterility* 43S–45S (1994).

Aoki, Bart, Chiang Peng Ngin, Bertha Mo, et al. "AIDS Prevention Model in Asian-American Communities." In *Primary Prevention of AIDS: Psychological Approaches.* V.M. Mays, G.W. Albee, and S.F. Schneider, eds. Newbury Park, CA: Sage, 1989.

Appiah-Kubi, Kofi. "Religion and Healing in an African Community: The Akan of Ghana." In *Healing and Restoring: Health and Medicine in the World's Religious Traditions.* L.E. Sullivan, ed. New York: Macmillan, 1989, pp. 203–24.

Bagley, Christopher, and Pierre Tremblay. "Suicidality Problems of Gay and Bisexual Males: Evidence from a Random Community Survey of 750 Men aged 18 to 27." In *Suicidal Behaviours in Adolescent and Adults: Taxonomy, Understanding and Prevention.* C. Bagley and R. Ramsay, eds. Brookfield, VT: Avebury, 1997.

Barsky, Arthur J. *Worried Sick: Our Troubled Quest for Wellness.* Boston, MA: Little,

Brown, 1988.

Beecher, Henry K. "The Powerful Placebo." 159 *Journal of the American Medical Association* 1602–6 (Dec. 24, 1955).

"Belgian Gay and Lesbian Youths More Likely to Attempt Suicide." *Outlines* (Chicago), Sept. 30, 1998, p. 10, col. 2.

Benson, Herbert, and David P. McCallie. "Angina Pectoris and the Placebo Effect." 300 *New England Journal of Medicine* 1424–29 (June 21, 1979).

Benson, Herbert, with Herbert Proctor. *Beyond the Relaxation Response*. New York: Berkeley, 1984.

Benson, Herbert, with Marg Stark. *Timeless Healing: The Power of Biology and Belief.* New York: Scribner, 1996.

Bhugra, D. "Doctors' Attitudes to Male Homosexuality: A Survey." 13 *Psychiatric Bulletin* 426–28 (1989).

Bickell, Nina A., Jo Anne Earp, Joanne M. Garrett, et al. "Gynecologists' Sex, Clinical Beliefs, and Hysterectomy Rates." 84 *American Journal of Public Health* 1649–52 (1994).

Bond, Charles F., Jr., Clarisse G. DiCandia, and John R. MacKinnon. "Responses to Violence in a Psychiatric Setting: The Role of the Patient's Race." 14 *Personality & Social Psychology Bulletin* 448–58 (1988).

The Boston Women's Health Book Collective. *Our Bodies, Ourselves—A Book by and for Women*. New York: Simon & Schuster, 1973.

Brewaeys, A., I. Ponjaert, E.V. Van Hall, et al. "Donor Insemination: Child Development and Family Functioning in Lesbian Mother Families." 12 *Human Reproduction* 1349–59 (June 6, 1997).

Broverman, Inge K., Donald M. Broverman, Frank E. Clarkson, et al. "Sex-Role Stereotypes and Clinical Judgments of Mental Health." 34 *Journal of Consulting & Clinical Psychology* 1–7 (Feb. 1970).

Burstin, Helen R., Stuart R. Lipsitz, and Troyen A. Brennan. "Socioeconomic Status and Risk for Substandard Medical Care." 268 *Journal of the American Medical Association* 2383–87 (Nov. 4, 1992).

Caelleigh, Addeane S. "Academic Medicine and the Issues of Aging." 72 *Academic Medicine* 835–38 (Oct. 1997).

Carrese, Joseph A., and Lorna A. Rhodes. "Western Bioethics on the Navajo Reservation: Benefit or Harm?" 274 *Journal of the American Medical Association* 826–29 (Sept. 13, 1995).

Chaimowitz, G.A. "Homophobia among Psychiatric Residents, Family Practice Residents and Psychiatric Faculty." 36 *Canadian Journal of Psychiatry* 206–9 (1991).

Chira, Susan. "Gay Parents Become Increasingly Visible." *N.Y. Times*, Sept. 30, 1993, Sec. A, p. 1.

Condor, Bob. "The Psychology of Compliance: Why Some People Don't Take Their Medicine." *Positively Aware*, March/April 1997, pp. 18–20.

Cooperstock, Ruth. "Sex Differences in the Use of Mood-Modifying Drugs: An Explanatory Model." 12 *Journal of Health & Social Behavior* 238–44 (Sept. 1971).

Cousins, Norman. *Head First: The Biology of Hope*. New York: E.P. Dutton, 1989.

Diamond, E. Grey, C. Frederick Kittle, and James E. Crockett. "Evaluation of Internal Mammary Artery Ligation and Sham Procedure in Angina Pectoris." 18 *Circulation* 712–13 (1958).

Dossey, Larry. *Healing Words: The Power of Prayer and the Practice of Medicine*. San Francisco: HarperSan Francisco, 1993.

———. *Meaning and Medicine: A Doctor's Tales of Breakthrough and Healing*. New York: Bantam, 1991.

Dunlap, David W. "Sperm Donor Is Awarded Standing as Girl's Father." *N.Y. Times*, Nov. 19, 1994, Sec 1., p. 27.

"FDA Approves 'Combivir' — Reduces Pill Regimens." *Outlines* (Chicago), Oct. 8, 1997, p. 13.

Feldman, Eric A., and Shohei Yonemoto. "Japan: AIDS as a 'Non-Issue'." In *AIDS in the Industrialized Democracies: Passions, Politics, and Policies*. D. Kirp and R. Bayer, eds. New Brunswick, NJ: Rutgers University Press, 1992, pp. 339–60.

Ferguson, Marilyn. *The Aquarian Conspiracy: Personal and Social Transformation in Our Time*. New York: G. P. Putnam, 1980.

Fielding, J.W.L., S.L. Fagg, B.G. Jones, et al. "An Interim Report of a Prospective, Randomized, Controlled Study of Adjuvant Chemotherapy in Operable Gastric Cancer: British Stomach Cancer Group." 7 *World Journal of Surgery* 390–99 (1983).

Fishman, Barbara L., Loretta Bobo, Kristy Kosub, et al. "Cultural Issues in Serving Minority Populations: Emphasis on Mexican Americans and African Americans." 306 *American Journal of the Medical Sciences* 160–66 (Sept. 1993).

Fitzpatrick, R., J. Dawson, M. Boulton, et al. "Perceptions of General Practice among Homosexual Men." 44 *British Journal of General Practice* 80–82 (1994).

Flaskerud, Jacquelyn H., and Li-tze Hu. "Racial/Ethnic Identity and Amount and Type of Psychiatric Treatment." 149 *American Journal of Psychiatry* 379–84 (March 1992).

Frank, Jerome. *Persuasion and Healing: A Comparative Study of Psychotherapy*, 3rd ed. Baltimore: Johns Hopkins University Press, 1991.

Geller, Stacie E., Lawton R. Burns, and David J. Brailler. "The Impact of Nonclinical Factors on Practice Variations: The Case of Hysterectomies." 30 *Health Services Research* 729–50 (Feb. 1996).

Goldston, David B., Maria Kovacs, D. Scott Obrosky, et al. "A Longitudinal Study of Life Events and Metabolic Control among Youths with Insulin-Dependent Diabetes Mellitus." 14 *Health Psychology* 409–14 (1995).

Goleman, Daniel. "Making Room on the Couch for Culture." *N.Y. Times*, Dec. 5, 1995, Sec. C (Science Times), pp. 1, 3.

Golombok, Susan, and Fiona Tasker. "Do Parents Influence the Sexual Orientation of Their Children? Findings From a Longitudinal Study of Lesbian Families." 32 *Developmental Psychology* 3–11 (Jan. 1996).

Greenberg, E.R., C.G. Chute, T. Stukel, et al. "Social and Economic Factors in the Choice of Lung Cancer Treatment: A Population-Based Study in Two Rural States." 318 *New England Journal of Medicine* 612–17 (1988).

Guo, Yuqui. "On Doing Yan Xin Qigong." See http://www.robelle.com/~dlo/qigong/articles/guo2.html.

Hackett, Thomas P., and Avery D. Weisman. "Predilection to Death: Death and Dying as a Psychiatric Problem." 23 *Psychosomatic Medicine* 232–56 (1961).

Hadley, Jack, Earl P. Steinberg, and Judith Feder. "Comparison of Uninsured and Privately Insured Hospital Patients: Condition on Admission, Resource Use, and Outcome." 265 *Journal of the American Medical Association* 374–79 (Jan. 16, 1991).

Harwood, Alan, ed. *Ethnicity and Medical Care*. Cambridge, MA: Harvard University Press, 1981.

Haynes, R. Brian, D. Wayne Taylor, and David L. Sackett, eds. *Compliance in Health Care*, 2nd ed. Baltimore: Johns Hopkins University Press, 1981.

"Health and Science: Physicians-Gay-Friendliness Is Contagious." *The Advocate*, Nov. 11, 1998, p. 18.

"Health Care Needs of Gay Men and Lesbians in the United States." 275 *Journal of the*

American Medical Association 1354–59 (May 1, 1996).

Helman, Cecil G. *Culture, Health and Illness: An Introduction for Health Professionals*, 2nd ed. London: Butterworth, 1990.

Horwitz, Ralph I., Catherine M. Viscoli, Lisa Berkman, et al. "Treatment Adherence and Risk of Death After a Myocardial Infarction." 336 *Lancet* 542–45 (Sept. 1, 1990).

Idler, E. "Self-Assessed Health and Mortality: A Review of Studies." In *International Review of Health Psychology,* Vol. 1, S. Maes, et al., eds. New York: John Wiley, 1992.

Ikemi, Yujiro, and Shunji Nakagawa. "A Psychosomatic Study of Contagion Dermatitis." 13 *Kyushu Journal of Medical Science* 335–50 (1962).

Jackson, Oscar J., and Waldense Nixon. "Medicine in the Black Community." 113 *California Medicine* 57–61 (October 1970).

Jacobsen, Frederick M. "Psychopharmacology." In *Women of Color: Integrating Ethnic and Gender Identity in Psychotherapy.* L. Comas-Díaz and L. Greene, eds. New York: Guilford Press, 1994, pp. 319–38.

Jhordan C. v. Mary K., 179 Cal. App. 3d 386 (1986).

Jones, James. *Bad Blood: The Tuskegee Syphilis Experiment.* New York: Free Press, 1981.

Justice, Blair. *Who Gets Sick: Thinking and Health.* Houston: Peak Press, 1987.

Kaufman, Barry Neil. *Happiness Is a Choice.* New York: Fawcett Columbine, 1991.

Kelly, Joan. "Sterilization and Civil Rights." 23 *Rights* 9–11 (1977).

Kirkpatrick, Martha. "Clinical Implications of Lesbian Mother Studies." In *Psychotherapy with Homosexual Men and Women: Integrated Identity Approaches for Clinical Practice.* E. Coleman, ed. New York: Haworth Press, 1988, pp. 201–11.

Krieger, Nancy, and Stephen Sidney. "Racial Discrimination and Blood Pressure: The CARDIA Study of Young Black and White Adults." 86 *American Journal of Public Health* 1370–78 (Oct. 1996).

Lewis, Dorothy Otnow, Shelley S. Shanok, Robert J. Cohen, et al. "Race Bias in the Diagnosis and Disposition of Violent Adolescents." 137 *American Journal of Psychiatry* 1211–16 (Oct. 1980).

Longino, Charles F., Jr. "Pressure from Our Aging Population Will Broaden Our Understanding of Medicine." 72 *Academic Medicine* 841–47 (Oct. 1997).

Loring, Marti, and Brian Powell. "Gender, Race, and DSM III: A Study of the Objectivity of Psychiatric Diagnostic Behavior." 29 *Journal of Health & Social Behavior* 1–22 (March 1988).

Lynch, James J. *The Language of the Heart: The Body's Response to Human Dialogue.* New York: Basic Books, 1985.

Maloney, Clarence, ed. *The Evil Eye.* New York: Columbia University Press, 1976.

Marieskind, Helen I. *Women in the Health System: Patients, Providers, and Program.* St. Louis: C. V. Mosby, 1980.

Maynard, Charles, Lloyd Fisher, and Eugene R. Passamani. "Blacks in the Coronary Artery Surgery Study (CASS): Race and Clinical Decision Making." 76 *American Journal of Public Health* 1446–48 (Dec. 1986).

Mechanic, David. "Development of Psychological Distress among Young Adults." 36 *Archives of General Psychiatry* 1233–39 (1979).

Minuchin, Salvador, Bernice L. Rosman, and Lester Baker. *Psychosomatic Families: Anorexia Nervosa in Context.* Cambridge, MA: Harvard University Press, 1978.

Murrell, N.L., R. Smith, G. Gill, et al. "Racism and Health Care Access: A Dialogue with Childbearing Women." 17 *Health Care for Women International* 149–59 (March/April 1996).

Ohnuki-Tierney, Emiko. "Health Care in Contemporary Japanese Religions." In *Healing and Restoring: Health and Medicine in the World's Religious Traditions.* L.E. Sullivan, ed. New York: Macmillan, 1989, pp. 59–87.

Olness, Karen, and Robert Ader. "Conditioning as an Adjunct in the Pharmacotherapy of Lupus Erythematosus," 13 *Journal of Developmental and Behavioral Pediatrics* 124–25 (April 1992).

Pachter, Lee M. "Culture and Clinical Care: Folk Illness Beliefs and Behaviors and Their Implications for Health Care Delivery." 271 *Journal of the American Medical Association* 690–94 (March 2, 1994).

"Patients Don't Always Reveal Their Sexual Orientation." 39 *American Medical News* 67 (May 6, 1996).

Pennebaker, James W. *The Psychology of Physical Symptoms.* New York: Springer-Verlag, 1982.

Pihl, R.O., Z. Segal, and L. Yankofsky. "The Effect of Alcohol and Placebo on Affective Reactions of Social Drinkers to a Procedure Designed to Induce Depressive Affect Anxiety and Hostility." 36 *Journal of Clinical Psychology* 337–42 (January 1980).

Plummer, K. "Gay and Lesbian Youth." In *Lesbian and Gay Youth in England.* G. Herdt, ed. New York: Harrington Park Press, 1989, pp. 193–223.

Porkert, Manfred, with Christian Ullmann. *Chinese Medicine.* Mark Howson, trans. New York: Henry Holt, 1982.

Reich, Warren Thomas, editor-in-chief. *Encyclopedia of Bioethics*, 2nd ed. New York: Macmillan, 1995.

Reichgott, M.J., and B.G. Simons-Mortons. "Strategies to Improve Compliance with Antihypertensive Therapy." 10 *Primary Care* 21–27 (1983).

"Reproductive Technologies." In *Encyclopedia of Bioethics*, 2nd ed., Vol. 4. New York: Macmillan, 1995.

Roberts, Alan H., Donald G. Kewman, Lisa Mercier, et al. "The Power of Nonspecific Effects in Healing: Implications for Psychosocial and Biologic Treatments." 13 *Clinical Psychology Review* 375–91 (1993).

Rosow, Irving. "Old Age: One Moral Dilemma for an Affluent Society." 2 *Gerontologist* 182–95 (1962).

Ross, Michael, and James M. Olson. "An Expectancy-Attribution Model of the Effects of Placebos." 88 *Psychological Review* 408–37 (1981).

Roter, Debra L., and Judith A. Hall. *Doctors Talking with Patients/Patients Talking with Doctors: Improving Communication in Medical Visits.* Westport, CT: Auburn House, 1993.

Roth, Robert T., and Judith Lerner. "Sex-Based Discrimination in the Mental Institutionalization of Women." 62 *California Law Review* 789–815 (May 1974).

Ruzek, Sheryl Burt. *The Women's Health Movement: Feminist Alternatives to Medical Control.* New York: Praeger, 1978.

Schiff, Robert L., David A. Ansell, James E. Schlosser, et al. "Transfers to a Public Hospital: A Prospective Study of 467 Patients." 314 *New England Journal of Medicine* 552–57 (Feb. 27, 1986).

Schoenfeld, David E., Lynda C. Malmrose, Dan G. Blazer, et al. "Self-Rated Health and Mortality in the High-Functioning Elderly: A Closer Look at Healthy Individuals." 49 *Journal of Gerontology* M109–15 (May 1994).

Scully, Diana, and Pauline Bart. "A Funny Thing Happened on the Way to the Orifice: Women in Gynecology Textbooks." 78 *American Journal of Sociology* 1045–50 (Jan. 1973).

Seaman, Barbara. *Free and Female.* New York: Fawcett, 1972.

Searching for Women: A Literature Review on Women with HIV/AIDS in the United States, 3rd ed. Boston: University of Massachusetts and Multicultural AIDS

Coalition, 1992.

Skinner v. Oklahoma, 316 U.S. 535 (1942).

Smith, Michael, Keh-Ming Lin, and Ricardo Mendoza. "'Nonbiological' Issues Affecting Psychopharmacotherapy: Cultural Considerations." In *Psychopharmacology and Psychology of Ethnicity*. K.M. Lin, R.E. Poland, and G. Kakasaki, eds. Washington: American Psychiatric Press, 1993, pp. 37–58.

Sontag, Susan. *Illness as Metaphor*. New York: Farrar, Strauss & Giroux, 1978.

Sorlie, Paul D., Norman J. Johnson, Eric Backlund, et al. "Mortality in the Uninsured Compared with That in Persons with Public and Private Health Insurance." 154 *Archives of Internal Medicine* 2409–16 (Nov. 14, 1994).

"Sterilization of Persons in Federally Assisted Programs of the Public Health Service." 42 C.F.R. § 50, 201 et seq. (1993).

"Sterilizations." 42 C.F.R. § 441.250 et seq. (1993).

Stevenson, Michael R., and Kathryn N. Black. "Parental Absence and Sex Role Development, A Meta-Analysis." 59 *Child Development* 793–814 (June 1988).

Stimson, Gerry V. "Obeying Doctor's Orders: A View from the Other Side." 8 *Social Science and Medicine* 97–104 (1974).

Strakowski, Stephen M., Heather S. Lonczak, Kenji W. Sax, et al. "The Effects of Race on Diagnosis and Disposition from a Psychiatric Emergency Service." 56 *Journal of Clinical Psychiatry* 101–7 (March 1995).

Tracy, John P. "Growing Up with Chronic Illness: The Experience of Growing Up with Cystic Fibrosis." 12 *Holistic Nursing Practice* 27–35 (1997).

Vitek v. Jones, 445 U.S. 480 (1980).

Voelker, Rebecca. "Nocebos Contribute to Host of Ills." 275 *Journal of the American Medical Association* 345, 347 (Feb. 7, 1996).

Wade, Jay C. "Institutional Racism: An Analysis of the Mental Health System." 63 *American Journal of Orthopsychiatry* 536–44 (1993).

Wade, Nicholas. "The Spin Doctors." *N.Y. Times Magazine*, Jan. 7, 1996, p. 16.

Wallick, Mollie M., Carl M. Cambre, and Mark H. Townsend. "How the Topic of Homosexuality Is Taught at U.S. Medical Schools." 67 *Academic Medicine* 601–3 (1992).

Weisman, Carol S. *Women's Health Care: Activist Traditions and Institutional Change*. Baltimore: Johns Hopkins University Press, 1998.

Wenneker, Mark B., Joel S. Weissman, and Arnold M. Epstein. "The Association of Payer with Utilization of Cardiac Procedures in Massachusetts." 264 *Journal of the American Medical Association* 1255–60 (Sept. 12, 1990).

Wheeler, Edwin O., Charles R. Williamson, and Mandel E. Cohen. "Heart Scare, Heart Surveys, and Iatrogenic Heart Disease." 167 *Journal of the American Medical Association* 1096–102 (1958).

Whitfield, LeRoy. "Black Plague: Whites Gain Some Reprieve from HIV, but African Americans Are Dying Faster than Ever." *Positively Aware*, September/October 1997, pp. 40–43, 45–46.

Wikler, Daniel, and Norma J. Wikler. "Turkey-Baster Babies: The Demedicalization of Artificial Insemination." 69 *Milbank Quarterly* 5–40 (1991).

Wray, Herbert. "Drug Death More Common in Uncommon Places." *Science News*, April 24, 1982, p. 279.

3

The Impact of Illness

INTRODUCTION: THE NATURE OF ILLNESS BEHAVIOR

Persons with comparable symptoms and limitations display extraordinary variation in how they perceive their health status, use medical care, and function in their social roles and work.

David Mechanic,
"Sociological Dimensions of Illness Behavior," p. 1211

The preceding statement illustrates that people who are ill display different reactions to their illness, including how they live and work. To some extent, these variations are described by medical sociologists when they define "illness behavior."

Unfortunately, illness behavior has often been described in negative terms; David Mechanic considers it the study of how sickness is used to seek potential advantages, to excuse failure and explain disappointment, to justify release from expected social roles and obligations, and to justify sympathy and dependence (ibid., p. 1208). This definition ignores the positive change in people's lives that illness may cause (e.g., some sick people become "independent" and do not seek to gain the sympathy of others). The positive response to illness that some sick people experience can be attributed to the peace of mind they acquire when they have accepted their condition and the honesty and increased clarity that they may develop when they recommit to their hopes and dreams.

The Struggle to Accept the Impact of Illness

It is often a struggle for many patients to accept the limitations of their chronic and terminal illnesses (see Hawkins, 1993). Limitations of such illnesses may include loss of or loss of function of various body parts. Bernie Siegel has said that many people die "rather than give up a part of their body" (Siegel, 1993, p. 83). But as the preceding statement poignantly suggests, much of the suffering caused by illness is perceptual or psychological—and medicine is not always equipped to help people reconstruct their lives.

According to the psychoanalyst Carl Jung, "We cannot change anything unless we accept it" (ibid., p. 24). To assist them to accept their illnesses, patients may be well served by health care professionals (HCPs) who can offer the support that can enable them to adapt to and ultimately live with their illnesses.

The ability to adapt to an illness may require one to "redefine" oneself, a form of readjusting self-concept or accepting that you're not the person you used to be (see Price, 1994, p. 182). As a result, ill persons may need to learn to find renewed meaning and purpose in their life.

A significant way human beings experience meaning in their lives is through their work. Our work enables us to be productive. But we must think about how we can find meaning in our lives when we are no longer able to work and be productive or creative. Viktor Frankl described a young man who courageously adapted to an inoperable spinal tumor that robbed him of many human functions (Frankl, 1957, pp. 51–52). He abandoned his profession because paralysis prevented him from working and, therefore, he could no longer be "creative." But he spent time in stimulating conversations with other patients— "entertaining them also, encouraging and consoling them. He devoted himself to reading good books, and especially to listening to good music on the radio. One day, however, he could no longer bear the pressure of the earphones, and his hands had become so paralyzed that he could no longer hold a book" (ibid.). This gentleman not only had to withdraw from creative values (required of his work) but from the "experiential values" described. Finally, he was forced to "retreat to attitudinal values . . . for he now set himself the role of adviser to his fellow sufferers, and in every way strove to be an exemplar to them. He bore his own suffering bravely" (ibid., p. 52).

Just because persons have accepted the limitations of an illness and the likelihood that it will cause their death does not mean that they must be resigned to having unproductive, unhappy, or unfulfilled lives. If we cannot be productive in the typical sense of being able to work, this does not mean that we cannot experience life as Frankl suggests. We can notice the beauty around us and counsel, console, encourage, and otherwise support family and friends. And even when we may no longer be able to "experience" life, we can maintain a positive attitude. Many of the survivors of prisons (and others experiencing deprivation in concentration camps or solitary confinement) have said that we must be aware of our capacity to choose our attitude and not feel defeated. With a positive attitude we can continue to create.[1] Because a positive attitude preserves our hopefulness, it enables us to feel connected to the human race and, consequently, often inspires us to make a contribution to our race.

The struggle to accept the impact of their illness may be eased for patients able to see the positive aspects of adversity—such as the new opportunities illness may create (see the section, "The Positive Impact of Illness").

The Consequences of Acceptance

Learning to accept one's condition, illness, or situation (e.g., whether one is homosexual or an alcoholic) often really frees one to live life. The following studies illustrate the consequence of accepting one's illness and situation:

- One study of patients who had acne for 15 or more years without relief concluded that several patients who were able to accept their acne rather than "resist" it with negative emotions found it cleared up within weeks (Ellerbroek, 1973).
- Patients with cancer who remained in denial about their illnesses were more likely to have poor prognoses than patients who accepted their illnesses (Ferguson, 1980, p. 252).[2]
- People with AIDS who accept their homosexuality and are "out" of the closet frequently have a better survival rate than those with AIDS who remain in the closet (Cole, Kemeny, Taylor, et al., 1996).

THE IMPACT OF ILLNESS ON FAMILIES

As mentioned in chapter 1, illness in one family member may significantly impact other members, particularly when they live together or are caregivers for a loved one. As a result, doctors may need to consider how the illness may impact a family's dynamics. Persons with chronic or terminal illnesses may impact their families dynamics in many ways:

- Family members who are caregivers for an ill person may find it stressful to meet the person's physical demands (such as feeding, lifting, making beds).
- Family members caring for ill parents, siblings, or relatives may resent the time devoted to their caregiving role even though they feel obligated to assume this role. Such "caregiving" tinged by resentment is likely to affect the sick person's care adversely.
- Family members who live with sick persons may be emotionally drained by routinely confronting the sick person's increasing limitations and varied emotional states. For example, some persons with illnesses may become resigned to die and may appear to "give up" on life, or they may become bored because they feel that their life no longer has meaning.
- Family members may be uncomfortable caring for a dying loved one because of their own fear of death and unresolved issues regarding death.

Physicians and others comprising a health care team (such as social workers and psychologists) can play an important role by providing relevant information to caregivers so that they understand some of the physical and psychological needs of the patient. Doctors should inform caregivers what to expect as the sick person's condition deteriorates or as the illness progresses.

Historically, some doctors have had difficulty relaying bad news to patients or their families. In a study of fourteen families in which one child had polio, doctors told only one family what to expect—so that they could avoid "scenes" with patients and "having to explain to and comfort them," tasks viewed as onerous and time-consuming (Davis, 1972).

Because of the impact of illness upon families, doctors should determine the state of the entire family's health, including the emotional and psychological well-being of the patient's spouse/significant other, siblings, and children (see Ellgring, Seiler, Perleth, et al., 1993). Caregivers who live in households where a sick person is depressed are at risk of development of depression themselves (Cousins, 1989, p. 23). And caregivers may also be at risk for a range of physical diseases; for example, caregivers of spouses diagnosed with Alzheimer's disease are at greater risk for immunological, neuroendocrine, cardiovascular, and metabolic problems (Scanlon, Vitalino, Ochs, et al., 1998).

THE IMPACT OF ILLNESS UPON INDIVIDUALS

Many studies have analyzed the traits of survivors who have withstood the assault of disease, trauma, or emotional distress (see Hirshberg & Barasch, 1995). Chart 3-1 details the most significant traits of survivors.

As already discussed, there is a psychological profile of the types of persons who best meet the challenges of illness. People often meet the challenge of illness in the following manner:

- By acquiring peace of mind, by loving oneself more and not necessarily seeking to be cured;
- By learning to accept their condition: as discussed in chapter 5, remarkable recoveries have been reported to occur in people who have accepted their illness and who pray to seek that God's will be done and to worship the glory of God; often, such persons do not pray to be cured (Dossey, 1993, p. 31);
- By developing an internal locus of control.

When persons with chronic and/or terminal conditions can acquire peace of mind, learn to accept their conditions, and become active participants in their lives (by taking steps or making decisions consistent with their hopes and dreams), they will become empowered by their illnesses. The nature of this empowerment is discussed further later.

Meeting the Challenges of Illness

Acquiring Peace of Mind. When sick and terminally ill persons gain peace of mind, they are often able to preserve, and sometimes to improve, the quality of life they had before becoming ill. Peace of mind occurs when we resolve issues in our lives that were a source of tension or trouble, whether that tension or trouble was caused by poor relationships or a job ill suited to our abilities and interests. Peace of mind also occurs when we live in the present and do not worry about or overfocus on the past and the future. In Western culture, it is a challenge to live in the present because the culture places a priority on being busy and on being productive. Peace of mind may also come when we embrace our uniqueness and do not feel compelled to conform to what others expect of us. Acquiring peace of mind is about learning to be happy.

We must be proactive to acquire peace of mind. We must make choices and take steps to make desired changes in our life. Someone else might make

---

Chart 3-1: Significant Traits of Survivors

Remain true to themselves during a crisis, a trait called *congruence* (Hirshberg & Barasch, 1995, p. 147)

Are often noncompliant with medical care (Hirshberg & Barasch, p. 147) (view of Spiegel)

Can express their needs and emotions (Siegel, 1989, p. 162; see Hirshberg & Barasch, p. 302)

Have a sense of personal responsibility for their health and "take charge" of their health care (Siegel, 1989, p. 162)

Have a sense of meaning and purpose in life (ibid.)

Have a feeling of fulfillment (Hirshberg & Barasch, p. 302) (view of Silberstein)

Often transform careers, marriages in concert with new-found purposes (ibid.)

Rediscover joy and creativity (ibid.)

Are flexible and have a wide array of resources upon which to draw (Siebert, 1993; see Siegel, 1986, pp. 163 et seq.)

Are resilient (Siebert, 1993)

Are adaptable (ibid.)

Make dietary changes (often becoming vegetarians) (Foster, 1988)

Accept their diagnosis

Do not perceive it as a death sentence (sometimes this requires individuals to reject the prognosis) (Hirshberg & Barasch, p. 201) (view of George Solomon)

Have a special healing relationship with either a spouse, a loved one, a support group, or a therapist (see Hirshberg & Barasch, p. 302) (view of Silberstein)

choices for us, but they will probably not reflect the authentic choices we would make for ourselves. As we make our own choices we will probably gain more self-respect. Acquiring peace of mind is closely associated with developing an internal locus of control.

Developing an Internal Locus of Control. Persons with an internal locus of control do not believe they are exclusively influenced by external factors but believe they can exert control over many things that will happen to them. Having an internal locus of control is not about the belief that we can change fate but about the idea that we can be active participants in our lives—that we need not wait to be "acted upon" by life. Psychologists estimate that 20 percent of the population have an inner locus of control (Siegel, 1986, p. 167).

Individuals who have an internal locus of control might also be considered to be "self-actualized." Abraham Maslow, who first used this term, defines *self-actualization* as

an episode, or a spurt in which the powers of the person come together in a particularly efficient and intensely enjoyable way, and in which he is more integrated and less split, more open for experience, more idiosyncratic, more perfectly expressive or spontaneous, more fully functioning, more creative, more humorous, more ego-transcending, more independent of his lower needs, etc. He becomes in these episodes more truly himself, more perfectly actualizing his potentialities, closer to the core of his Being, more fully human. (Maslow, 1968, p. 97)

Other qualities of the self-actualized person are detailed in Chart 3-2. Maslow estimated that less than 1 percent of adults are self-actualized (ibid., p. 204).[3]

Many cultural and religious views support people's notions that they do not control some of the things that may happen to them. Some religious people who believe in reincarnation also believe that a person's "path" in this life is fixed: that some persons are destined to be poor or to suffer, and, therefore, they can (and should) do little to alter their lot (Green, 1990; Little, 1990).

EXTERNAL FACTORS THAT IMPACT THE PATIENT'S HEALTH

Health care professionals must remain sensitive to the patient as a whole person. They must not focus on the patient's medical condition to the exclusion of considering the patient's mental health or other sociopsychological issues with which the patient is concerned. In order for HCPs to focus on patients, they must consider the nature of their environment, support network, and the effects of society's views about illness on them (i.e., are patients overwhelmed by the stigma associated with their illness?).

The Nature of the Patient's Environment

Patients' relationships to their environment have long been known to influence health (see Moorman, 1950). Immigrants removed from their countries of origin

---

Chart 3-2: Qualities of Self-Actualized Persons

Creativity	Take Time for Solitude
No Fear of Ridicule	Superior Perception of Reality
No Fear of the Unknown	Increased Self-Acceptance
No Need for Certainty	Tolerant—Accepting of Others
Positive Self-Valuation	Resists Tendency to Generalize
Resourceful Learners	Looks at the Whole Person
Drive toward Autonomy	Democratic Character Structure
Instinct to Be Productive	Capable of Righteous Indignation
Believe Struggle Is Meaningful	Spontaneous
Courage	Have More Peak Experiences
Enhanced Emotional Reactions	Improved Interpersonal Relations
Fraught with Polarities	Selfish and Unselfish
Self Trust (Individuals Have Staying Power in Times of Uncertainty)	Optimistic (Supports Faith in Ourselves and Abilities)

Sources: Maslow, Abraham H., *Toward a Psychology of Being,* 2nd ed. (Princeton, NJ: D. Van Nostrand, 1968); Sinetar, Marsha, *Living Happily Ever After: Creating Trust, Luck and Joy* (New York: Villard, 1990).

(e.g., the Hmong refugees from Laos) or Native Americans removed from their original lands have experienced adverse health consequences, including death, after such dislocation (Benson with Stark, 1996, p. 84–86 [Hmong refugees]; Justice, 1987, pp. 3–4; Moorman, 1950 [Native Americans]). When patients perceive their new environment as a threat, because it is different or even hostile, they may be unable to adjust to it. A combination of the feelings of hopelessness, despair, frustration, and stress may cause sickness and/or death.

The Patient's Support Network

The type of and extent of support the patient receives are also related to the state of the patient's health. Consider the following examples illustrating the relationship between increased life expectancy and support:

- As already mentioned, women with metastatic breast cancer who joined support groups lived twice as long as those who received only medical care (Spiegel, Bloom, Kraemer, et al., 1989).
- Persons receiving extensive support from members of their community also have a reduced mortality rate even when they engaged in unhealthy behavior like smoking, drinking, and not exercising (Bruhn & Wolf, 1979).
- Individuals (particularly husbands) who lose the companionship and support of their spouses through death have increased mortality rates (Parkes, Benjamin, & Fitzgerald, 1969).

Doctors should be aware that before entering the health care or hospital setting, some patients may have been abandoned or experienced discrimination. For example, patients with AIDS may have been abandoned by their families, fired from their jobs, denied coverage by their insurance companies; they may have faced harassment by and received rude calls from a creditor, and felt disrespect (or even humiliation) when seeking public benefits from bureaucrats in government agencies. These external factors may impose more stress on them than that imposed by their disease. The patient may have bona fide reasons for being frustrated, angry, lonely, dejected, and hopeless.

Patients also receive support from their pets. Pets are known to affect the physiological processes and health of their owners. Studies show that although the blood pressure of pet owners rose significantly when they spoke with an experimenter, their blood pressure either decreased or remained the same when they spoke with their pets (Lynch, 1985, p. 155). Of patients with cardiovascular disease discharged from a hospital, 28 percent died within one year if they did not own a pet, but only 6 percent of the pet owners died during the same period (Friedmann, Katcher, Lynch, et al., 1980).

Many factors that provide support in our lives, from intimate relationships to pets, also seem to provide our lives with meaning and purpose. People often feel hopeless when the sense of meaning and purpose is stripped from their lives, and, as a result, they may have a greater risk of mortality.

Society's Views about Illness

Patients with illnesses may need to face the public perception that they are "contaminated" or even "morally polluted." Society's perception of illness may impact patients' self-perception and may cause them to feel shame or guilt. Astoundingly, these feelings are associated with increased morbidity and mortality rates (see Cole, Kemeny, Taylor, et al., 1996). As already noted, gay men with AIDS who are not out of the closet have a higher mortality rate than those who are able to acknowledge and speak about their homosexuality (ibid.); this may be due to the fact that the former group feels shame and stigma because they are gay and because they have AIDS, whereas the latter group has been able to accept who they are.

Many writers have discussed the public's perception that persons with certain diseases are "contaminated" (i.e., the belief that a certain kind of person is likely to become ill) (Musto, 1988, p. 77) or even "morally polluted" (see Sontag, 1978). Throughout history, the public perceived many diseases to reflect the social inferiority of those affected or thought that those affected were immoral and contracted disease because of their immorality (see Rosenberg, 1988). At one time, those who contracted cholera were believed to comprise "the dirty, the gluttonous, and the poorly nourished" (ibid., p. 18).

Physicians have even been caught up in this "moralizing" (ibid., p. 22). Some physicians advised that sexual moderation and temperance were critical to the control of cholera (Risse, 1988, pp. 41, 46).

The advancement of science and the existence of the germ theory of disease have not altered public perceptions that disease affects people who are "bad" or sinful or that people with diseases are contaminated. People with AIDS have been abandoned by their churches or refused church membership (Hilts, 1992), and some people with cancer cannot sell their houses because prospective purchasers will not buy a home that has been inhabited by a person with cancer (see Photopulos, 1991, p. 112). This and other types of discrimination obviously put a certain stress on sick patients who are conformists and who seek social approval in order to "function" effectively.

THE POSITIVE IMPACT OF ILLNESS

> We must all become familiar with the thought of death if we want to grow into really good people. . . . Thinking about death produces love for life.
>
> Albert Schweitzer
> quoted in Kushner,
> *How Good Do We Have to Be?* p. 157

Many people with chronic or terminal illnesses, perceived by the general public to be without hope, have actually been empowered by their illness and have become more productive (see Hawkins, 1993), repaired damaged relationships (or cut their losses and moved on to more wholesome relationships), and learned to live their lives and, consequently, learned to be who they are and pursue their dreams (they no longer live vicariously through others). People who have learned to speak honestly with others

- often experience a freedom unique among the living; this sense of freedom is very empowering.
- do not feel as though they are living a lie; they feel as though they are "authentic" persons.
- do not have relationships with people who do not accept them as they are.

Introduction: The Nature of Empowerment for Persons with Illnesses

The empowerment many people experience because of their illnesses may consist of the following:

- Attaining spiritual rebirth or awareness (see ibid.).
- Achieving greater fulfillment in their relationships and more honest relations with their families.
- Making changes in their work-related goals and objectives: These changes occur when persons become active participants in their lives. They are achieved with the clarity, focus, and determination that often accompany terminal and chronic illness.
- Appreciating the personal growth associated with reflection.
- Valuing present moments and, therefore, attempting to extract as much joy out of a day as possible: Our culture, which causes us to focus on our accomplishments, does not encourage us to appreciate our journey toward those accomplishments (see Benson with Stark, 1996, p. 263).

It has been said that death concentrates the mind wonderfully (Storr, 1988, p. 169). When people appreciate that their time is limited, they often proceed to use their time more effectively. They learn to do what they have always yearned to do.

Becoming More Spiritually Aware

The physician Herbert Benson has noted that after a relaxation response, 25 percent of patients tend to be more spiritual (Benson with Stark, 1996, p. 155). People with terminal illnesses often become more spiritually aware as they turn their thoughts inward to contemplate what they want to do with their remaining time. Furthermore, once they learn to accept their condition or diagnosis, they frequently become more calm. This state of calm enables them to be more aware and enhances the ability to be contemplative—contemplation incubates insight and enables creativity (ibid., p. 278). Spiritual awareness is also associated with peace of mind and a state of being calm.

Being in Touch with One's Expectations Regarding Life and Work

When patients become aware that illness may limit their time on earth, they often want their lives to reflect much more personal and professional (or work-related) meaning. They want their lives to stand for something because they may want to be remembered, to make a contribution to society (see Huisman, 1997),[4] and to have richer relationships. They no longer want to focus on trivia or things that to them are not meaningful.

Because of their awareness of their limited time, people with chronic and terminal illnesses often carefully develop a list of priorities, things that are important to them: things to accomplish and goals to achieve. To develop goals, people need to determine what is important to them or to consider how they may wish to be remembered. The author Stephen Covey suggests that people write their own obituaries—then they will know how they would like to be remembered (Covey, 1990, p. 98).

Being More Honest about One's Needs and Emotions

Freed from the bonds of convention and the fear of what others may think, the mind responds with new solutions, new goals, and an awareness that beauty and peace come from within.

Bernie S. Siegel,
Love, Medicine and Miracles, p. 167

Most people have a great deal of difficulty expressing their needs and emotions because much human behavior is designed to seek the approval of others. In other words, because they feel the ridicule, scorn, or isolation from others, they do not truthfully offer their opinions or pursue their preferred work. They may tell you, perhaps, what they think you want to hear and obtain work that may meet with your approval. This amounts to living someone else's life rather than their own. Although such persons may appear to be independent of others, they are actually quite dependent upon them, needing approval to sustain their self-concept.

One study estimated that only 10–20 percent of people would refuse to do a favor for a friend if they did not want to do it (Siegel, 1989, pp. 162–63). Oddly enough, this ability to say no has been associated with long-term survival. When people decide to live their lives authentically and be honest with others, they also have the capacity to empower others with honesty. One of the greatest consequences of being honest and sharing feelings with others is the exhilaration of being free to live your life. The persons with whom you are honest may not feel so liberated: they may cling to their interpretation of reality. Expressing feelings may also speed rehabilitation from injury (Siegel, 1986, p. 104) and cause less stress and fewer psychological problems (ibid.).

Increased Clarity

Terminal illness often causes enhanced clarity. This is probably the result of prioritizing projects and work; the increased calm that patients may experience is related to the peace of mind they may attain and their increased commitment to the projects they consider high-priority. This commitment often increases their determination to see the project to completion. When projects are pursued with determination, focus and concentration inevitably follow. With a clear sense of mission in life and a sense of priorities, it is much easier to learn how to fill the day with joy and important work.

The need for ill persons to redefine themselves is critical to their ability to restructure their time. If people can no longer work, their time is no longer structured by their job-related tasks. They must redefine their relationship to time and determine what they want to accomplish with the time available to them.

Having a formal job is almost always considered important by members of society at large. When people lose their jobs, through either sickness or retirement, they sometimes feel less important, because in their minds they are not making valuable contributions to society. People who are sick or retired, therefore, need to learn how to use their time so that they can still feel valued. They have to come up with their own ideas and define meaningful work for themselves, as opposed to having employers tell them what is important. This is, in short, what it means to become an active participant in your life because you have to create a plan of action to preserve your self-worth and self-esteem.

Focusing on Giving

> Living with the knowledge that we're going to die someday means that we may choose to give something to the world.
>
> Bernie S. Siegel,
> *Love, Medicine and Miracles*, p. 169

Other authors have echoed Dr. Bernie Siegel's sentiments of our quite human tendency to want to leave a legacy and to want our life to have "mattered" (Huisman, 1997; Kushner, 1986, p. 20). We do not have to leave tangible things behind in order to leave a legacy. We may act as role models, and, by the way we act, we may show others our value system. We may share our love with others and show them respect. These feelings and values, when shared with others, may empower them.

Learning to Experience Happiness

If one accepts the Dalai Lama's supposition that the purpose of life is to be happy, then it seems reasonable to assume that persons who really live their life will be happy.[5] We will first examine some of the most common definitions of happiness and then consider how these definitions relate to the ability to live one's life.

Among typical definitions of happiness are the following:

- "The true joy in life [is] being used for a purpose recognized by yourself as a mighty one" (George Bernard Shaw, 1903).
- Happiness is about holding fast to the principles from which our desires and actions spring (Smith, 1899, p. 112 quoting Marcus Aurelius).[6]
- "Happiness isn't something that depends on our surroundings. It's something we make inside ourselves" (Corrietan Boom) (see Humphries, 1980, p. 88).
- "The only ones among you who will be really happy are those who will have sought and found how to serve" (Albert Schweitzer) (see Bryant, 1991, p. 150).
- "Happiness includes the ability to accept what you are and know that it isn't so bad" (Roberta Jean Bryant) (ibid., p. 88).

These definitions not only highlight some of the major themes about the nature of happiness but illustrate that we can only attain happiness through indirect, not direct, means. They point out that happiness comes to those

- whose life is rich in meaning and purpose,
- who have values and principles and who walk their talk,
- whose values and principles compel them to serve others,
- who develop their inner selves, and
- who learn the power of acceptance.

Taking Personal Responsibility for One's Health

Taking personal responsibility for one's health includes exercising control over factors that one can control such as one's diet (see Foster, 1988)[7] and making decisions in concert with one's doctor (discussed more extensively in chapter 6). It is quite possible that the dietary changes one may make will not do anything to make one healthier. But the belief that they are worthwhile or positive changes, and the measure of control over one's wellness that they enable patients to feel, may elicit their own independent benefits.

THE NEGATIVE IMPACT OF ILLNESS

Long-term illness is often associated with eight fears: fear of the loss of control, fear of the loss of self-image, fear of dependency, fear of stigma, fear of abandonment, fear of expressing anger, fear of isolation, and fear of death (Pollin & Golant, 1994). Illness may negatively impact people when it jeopardizes their ability to maintain their self-esteem—they may not feel as valuable, important, or worthy of being loved as they once were. Loss of one's job through illness may threaten one's self-esteem, particularly as persons become dependent upon others and lose their ability to be productive. As already discussed, the ability to be productive and to have something to show for one's efforts is highly prized in American society. In fact, Americans probably cannot even enjoy their leisure time unless they are producing. Although chronic illness seems to take away some of our choices, we must be aware that often we retain the ability to make other choices. Coping with chronic or terminal illness is often about redefining oneself and learning to take in stride the inevitable life changes that are to follow. Last, dying of a chronic or terminal illness is often viewed as tragic. But if we viewed death as a natural life event and as natural as birth itself, we might not see it as tragic. Many have come not to view death as tragic, but rather to view as tragic that many people have never really lived their lives. In the eyes of Dr. Arthur J. Barsky, "[W]e are pursuing perfect health and yet living all the while like invalids" (Barsky, 1988, p. 19). Sometimes such people come to the end of their lives only to realize that they have never lived.

Financial Dependence

When people with chronic or terminal illnesses become unable to work, loss of the income from full-time employment may cause them to become financially dependent upon others. Their reduced income may necessitate a reduction in their standard of living.

Loss of Personal Independence

Persons with illnesses and disabilities have much in common with the elderly. Sometimes the well-intentioned family members of such persons make decisions for them even though they remain fully capable of making their own. Such family members do not always see the important distinction between offering compassion and support and taking away people's ability to remain independent or to exert control over their destiny. Health care professionals must be sensitive to ill people's desires to make decisions regarding the "nature of their destiny," particularly their right to make health-related decisions as long as they remain competent and choose to do so.

Illness often renders us unable to do things we may have typically done for ourselves. We may look upon our inability to be independent, autonomous, and in control of the detail of our daily lives as if it were a curse. But we may fail to realize that we may gain something when we lose control: we may learn how to accept the love and concern of others, for illness puts us on the receiving—not the giving—end.

Changing Relationships

Illness may result in some changed relationships with spouses, friends, and family members. Sexual and intimate relationships may also be changed, particularly in illnesses that may make men impotent or illnesses such as AIDS (see Rabkin, Remien, Katoff, et al., 1993 [AIDS]). At least 90 percent of gay men with AIDS who were long-term survivors and considered to be coping well with their illness reported widespread dissatisfaction with their sex lives—this contributed to a sense of loneliness and lack of joy in life (ibid.).

Social Isolation

The social isolation that may accompany illness is often associated with the fear the living may have of facing issues of disability and death. Illness may rob us of many things—appearance, stamina, and energy to complete simple tasks. But as also emphasized throughout this chapter, illness may provide us with the opportunity for much emotional growth. It may be awkward for many healthy persons to communicate with those who have disabilities and who are terminally ill. In communicating with the terminally ill, the healthy should remember that the terminally ill person is not yet dead. As Bernie Siegel says, patients are either alive or dead (Siegel, 1986, p. 44). While they are living, persons with terminal illnesses should be treated with the respect we often accord to the healthy.

CHAPTER SUMMARY

Individuals with a sickness or disease have varying responses to being ill. Additionally, caregivers, friends, and family members of those who are ill similarly have varied responses to the person who is sick. Doctors should not only be cognizant of treating their patients who are sick, but be aware of the many needs of caregivers and others who are in regular contact with the patient. The psychological health of caregivers may be greatly affected by their loved one who is sick.

Patients can often successfully meet the challenges of illness by acquiring peace of mind, accepting their conditions, and developing an internal locus of control. They can acquire peace of mind and decrease their worries, focus on their present moments, explore their uniqueness without feeling the pressures for conformity, and resolve issues that were previously a source of tension (e.g., one can strive to repair relationships). But to acquire peace of mind, patients must be proactive. Developing an internal locus of control will support proactivity—the ability to make decisions consistent with one's hopes and dreams.

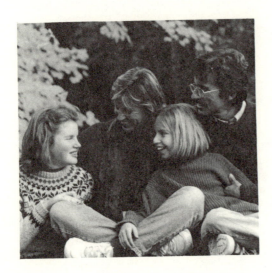

AN INTERVIEW WITH PAULINE BANDUCCI

I am 42 years old. My daughter Julia was diagnosed with autism at age four although when she was 18 months old I knew that she was not developing normally. She pushed, hit and bit children and adults, screamed day and night, did not smile or laugh, could not speak, and was obsessed with food. She even scavenged in trash cans to find food.

Persons with autism often use repetitious behaviors to withdraw from a world they find confusing. Because a person's behavior is often unpredictable, persons with autism seem to prefer playing with objects because they are "predictable" (they do not get angry or sad). It has been shown that the brains of persons with autism overproduce serotonin, a neurotransmitter associated with good moods. It is quite possible that autistic individuals may feel that they do not really need to have relationships with people because they are already happy.

Julia actually had severe autism. The doctors whom my spouse and I consulted did not provide much encouragement regarding the treatment outcomes of traditional medicine. We were told that Julia's violent behavior would get worse as she became an adult and that she would never really be able to be in public (like going to church or to the movies) because of the sounds she made. I had heard of The Option Institute in Sheffield, Massachusetts, and their work with the families of "special needs" children.

The staff of The Option Institute taught me how to calm down and not necessarily judge Julia's behavior as "bad." More specifically, they taught me how to use my daughter's passions for sound and food to both her and to my advantage. We used Julia's passion for sound to learn the sounds of the animal kingdom: from dinosaurs to cats. Julia gradually learned to speak and to read because of her love of sound. To indulge her passion for food, we played "hide and seek" to create fun games involving food. These games enabled Julia to connect with me. As I entered her world with sincerity and enthusiasm, we both began to change.

Julia is now 15 years old and still has autism. She smiles, laughs, and no longer exhibits any violent behavior. She grooms and bathes herself and helps with the laundry and dishes. She no longer has an obsession with food. She reads books and attends school although she is in a sixth grade classroom. I've seen Julia progress year by year.

I believe children with autism have many things to teach us. Children with autism don't have the beliefs (including prejudices) about people that many of us acquire as we grow up. Adults filter everything we perceive in the world through our belief system. When I changed my original beliefs about my daughter, that she was a "terrible tragedy" or that "I couldn't deal with her," I was able to first accept and then to love her unconditionally.

In June 1996, I became a staff member at The Option Institute. Several families with children with autism who had come to The Option Institute because of their children with autism have reported to us that their children no longer have autism. Apparently the physicians for these children also find no further evidence of autism. At the Institute, we believe that if children are motivated enough, they are able to change their behaviors (and we believe that this changed behavior is accompanied by changes in brain tissue and chemistry).

Although I no longer work at The Option Institute, I believe that, because I've applied what I learned there, I've become an authentic person: saying what I think and meaning what I say. I've been able to apply what I've learned about my relationship with my daughter to my relationship with my husband. In short, the less judgmental I become about what I believe are his "faults," the more accepting and loving I become of him.

NOTES

1. Frankl's case scenario suggests that when we must rely on our "attitudinal" values, we have lost our ability to be "creative." Although physical limitations may not enable us to write and to paint, this author believes that our attitudes may enable us to create in our minds.

2. This information is consistent with studies that show that women with breast cancer in support groups survive twice as long as women who do not participate in such support groups (Spiegel, Bloom, Kraemer, et al., 1989). Obviously, women who discuss with each other the effects of cancer on their lives and the ways in which cancer has changed their perspectives cannot remain in denial of their illness.

3. Maslow has offered his perspective as to why so few adults are self-actualizing: He says that "growth" has many intrinsic pains (Maslow, 1968, p. 204). He continues,

Each step forward is a step into the unfamiliar and is possibly dangerous. It also means giving up something familiar and good and satisfying. It frequently means a parting and a separation, even a kind of death prior to rebirth, with consequent nostalgia, fear, loneliness and mourning. It also often means giving up a simpler and less effortful life, in exchange for a more demanding, more responsible, more difficult life. Growth forward *is in spite* of these losses and therefore requires courage, will, choice, and strength in the individual, as well as protection, permission, and encouragement from the environment, especially for the child. (emphasis in original) (ibid.)

4. At least for people with AIDS, one author suggests that men seek to be "known to others before they die"—leaving a legacy of accomplishment (Huisman, 1997). Women, however, find it important to participate in AIDS education and prevention. The author notes that men tend to disclose their HIV status to connect with others. But women who feel the shame and stigma associated with HIV/AIDS are unlikely to disclose their condition to others except to other women with AIDS who can serve as role models.

5. In this author's opinion there are many levels of happiness. Those who are most happy may be joyful, ecstatic, or exhilarated. Those who are less happy might be content or satisfied.

6. Marcus Aurelius's view that happiness revolves around having principles that relate to what is good is illustrated by the following quote:

[Happiness is to be found] in doing what human nature requires. How shall you do this? By holding fast to the principles from which our desires and actions spring. What principles? Those that relate to good and evil: that nothing is truly good for a man which does not make him just, temperate, courageous, and free; and that nothing can be evil for a man which gives him not the contrary dispositions. (Smith, 1899, p. 112)

7. A review of 200 cases of remarkable recoveries from cancer found that 88 percent of recovered persons made substantial dietary changes, usually of a "strict vegetarian nature" (Foster, 1988).

SUGGESTED READING

Hawkins, Anne Hunsaker. *Reconstructing Illness: Studies in Pathography*. West Lafayette, IN: Purdue University Press, 1993.

REFERENCES

Barsky, Arthur J. *Worried Sick: Our Troubled Quest for Wellness*. Boston: Little, Brown, 1988.

Benson, Herbert, with Marg Stark. *Timeless Healing: The Power of Biology and Belief*. New York: Scribner, 1996.

Bruhn, John G., and Stewart Wolf. *The Roseto Story: An Anatomy of Health*. New York: Harper & Row, 1979.

Bryant, Roberta Jean. *Stop Improving Yourself and Start Living*. San Rafael, CA: New World Library, 1991.

Cole, Steve W., Margaret E. Kemeny, Shelley E. Taylor, et al. "Accelerated Course of Human Immunodeficiency Virus Infection in Gay Men Who Conceal Their Homosexual Identity." 58 *Psychosomatic Medicine* 219–31 (May 1996).

Cousins, Norman. *Head First: The Biology of Hope*. New York: E. P. Dutton, 1989.

Covey, Stephen. *The Seven Habits of Highly Effective People*. New York: Fireside/Simon & Schuster, 1990.

Davis, Fred. "Uncertainty in Medical Prognosis, Clinical and Functional." In *Medical Men and Their Work: A Sociological Reader*. E. Friedson and J. Lorber, eds. Chicago: Aldine Atherton, 1972, pp. 239–48.

Dossey, Larry. *Healing Words: The Power of Prayer and the Practice of Medicine*. San Francisco: HarperSan Francisco, 1993.

Ellerbroek, Wallace E. "Hypotheses Toward a Unified Field Theory of Human Behavior with Clinical Application to Acne Vulgaris." 16 *Perspectives in Biology and Medicine* 240–62 (Winter 1973).

Ellgring, H., S. Seiler, B. Perleth, et al. "Psychosocial Aspects of Parkinson's." 43 *Neurology* (12 Suppl. 6) S41–44 (Dec. 1993).

Ferguson, Marilyn. *The Aquarian Conspiracy: Personal and Social Transformation in Our Time*. New York: G. P. Putnam, 1980.

Foster, Harold. "Lifestyle Changes and the 'Spontaneous' Regression of Cancer." 10 *International Journal of Biosocial Research* 17–33 (1988).

Frankl, Viktor. *The Doctor and the Soul*. New York: Alfred Knopf, 1957.

Friedmann, Erika, Aaron H. Katcher, James J. Lynch, et al. "Animal Companions and One-Year Survival of Patients after Discharge from a Coronary Care Unit." 95 *Public Health Reports* 307–12 (1980).

Green, Ronald M. "Buddhist Economic Ethics: A Theoretical Approach." In *Ethics, Wealth, and Salvation: A Study in Buddhist Social Ethics*. R.F. Sizemore and D.K. Swearer, eds. Columbia: University of South Carolina Press, 1990.

Hawkins, Anne Hunsaker. *Reconstructing Illness: Studies in Pathography*. West Lafayette, IN: Purdue University Press, 1993.

Hilts, Philip J. "Touched by AIDS: Minister Finds Door Shut." *N.Y. Times*, Sept. 8, 1992, p. 1.

Hirshberg, Caryle, and Marc Ian Barasch. *Remarkable Recovery: What Extraordinary Healings Tell Us about Getting Well and Staying Well*. New York: Riverhead Books, 1995.

Huisman, Mark J. "Over Sensibilities: The Art of Transcending the Here and Now." *POZ*, April 1997, p. 46.

Humphries, Jackie. *All the Things You Aren't Yet*. Waco, TX: World Books, 1980.

Justice, Blair. *Who Gets Sick: Thinking and Health*. Houston: Peak Press, 1987.

Kushner, Harold. *How Good Do We Have to Be? A New Understanding of Guilt and Forgiveness*. Boston: Little, Brown, 1996.

———. *When All You've Ever Wanted Isn't Enough*. New York: Summit Books, 1986.

72 Producing Patient-Centered Health Care

Little, David. "Ethical Analysis and Wealth in Theravada Buddhism: A Response to Frank Reynolds." In *Ethics, Wealth, and Salvation: A Study in Buddhist Social Ethics.* R.F. Sizemore and D.K. Swearer, eds. Columbia: University of South Carolina Press, 1990.

Lynch, James J. *The Language of the Heart: The Body's Response to Human Dialogue.* New York: Basic Books, 1985.

Maslow, Abraham. *Toward a Psychology of Being*, 2nd ed. Princeton, NJ: D. Van Nostrand, 1968.

Mechanic, David. "Sociological Dimensions of Illness Behavior." 41 *Social Science and Medicine* 1207–16 (1995).

Moorman, Lewis J. "Tuberculosis on the Navajo Reservation." 61 *American Review of Tuberculosis* 586–91 (1950).

Musto, David F. "Quarantine and the Problem of AIDS." In *AIDS: The Burden of History.* E. Fee and D. Fox, eds. Berkeley: University of California Press, 1988, pp. 67–85.

Parkes, C. Murray, B. Benjamin, and R.G. Fitzgerald. "Broken Heart: A Statistical Study of Increased Mortality among Widowers." 1 *British Medical Journal* 740–43 (March 22, 1969).

Photopulos, Georgia. "Experiences in Cancer: Bridging the Gap Between Patients and Professionals." In *Health and Faith: Medical, Psychological and Religious Dimensions.* J.T. Chirban, ed. Lanham, MD: University Press of America, 1991, pp. 105–14.

Pollin, Irene, with Susan K. Golant. *Taking Charge: Overcoming the Challenge of Long-Term Illness.* New York: Times Books, 1994.

Price, Reynolds. *A Whole New Life.* New York: Atheneum, 1994.

Rabkin, Judith G., Robert H. Remien, L. S. Katoff, et al. "Resilience in Adversity among Long-Term Survivors of AIDS." 44 *Hospital and Community Psychiatry* 162–67 (1993).

Risse, Guenter B. "Epidemics and History: Ecological Perspectives and Social Responses." In *AIDS: The Burden of History.* E. Fee and D. Fox, eds. Berkeley: University of California Press, 1988, pp. 33–66.

Rosenberg, Charles. "Disease and Social Order in America: Perceptions and Expectations." In *AIDS: The Burden of History.* E. Fee and D. Fox, eds. Berkeley: University of California Press, 1988, pp. 12–32.

Scanlon, James M., Peter P. Vitaliano, Hans Ochs, et al. "CD4 and CD8 Counts Are Associated with Interactions of Gender and Psychosocial Stress." 60 *Psychosomatic Medicine* 644–53 (1998).

Shaw, George Bernard. *Man and Superman, a Comedy and a Philosophy.* New York: Bretano's, [c. 1903].

Siebert, Al. *The Survivor Personality.* Portland, OR: Practical Psychology Press, 1993.

Siegel, Bernie S. *How to Live Between Office Visits: A Guide to Life, Love and Health.* New York: HarperCollins, 1993.

———. *Love, Medicine and Miracles: Lessons Learned about Self-Healing from a Surgeon's Experience with Exceptional Patients.* New York: Harper & Row, 1986.

———. *Peace, Love and Healing: Bodymind Communication and the Path to Self-Healing: An Exploration.* New York: Harper & Row, 1989.

Sinetar, Marsha. *Living Happily Ever After: Creating Trust, Luck, and Joy.* New York: Villard, 1990.

Smith, Benjamin, trans. *Selections from the Meditations of Marcus Aurelius.* New York: The Century Co., 1899.

Sontag, Susan. *Illness as Metaphor.* New York: Farrar, Straus & Giroux, 1978.

Spiegel, David, Joan R. Bloom, Helena C. Kraemer, et al. "Effects of Psychosocial

Treatment on Survival of Patients with Metastatic Breast Cancer." *Lancet* 888–91 (Oct. 15, 1989).

Storr, Anthony. *Solitude: A Return to the Self.* New York: Free Press, 1988.

4

The Role of Emotions and Personality in Health

INTRODUCTION

> Man is a speck of reason in an ocean of emotion.

William James
quoted in Rogers,
On Becoming a Person, p. 312

Psychologists and philosophers have quibbled over the meaning of emotions for over a century (Goleman, 1995, p. 289). And researchers cannot agree as to which emotions are primary. Because there are facial expressions for fear, anger, sadness, and enjoyment, and because these expressions are recognized by people in cultures around the world, some have said these expressions indicate the "core emotions" (ibid., p. 290). A list of common emotions is provided in Chart 4-1.

Chart 4-1: The Emotions

Anger (aggravation; frustration)	Hate
Boredom	Hope
Contentment	Jealousy
Despair	Joy
Envy	Loneliness
Fear	Resentment
Forgiveness	Revenge
Happiness	Sadness

The emotions generally include impulses to act (ibid., p. 6). These impulses can be affected by interaction with the intellect and can certainly be constructive or destructive. Our emotions reflect and are influenced by

- our moods (happy versus sad),
- our perceptions of the behavior or motivations of others (do we see them as a threat?),
- ways in which we experience our free time or time alone (are we lonely or bored?),
- our view of the purpose of life (are we fearful, happy, or sad?), and
- our perception of ourselves in relation to others and to society. For example, shame and guilt are a reaction to how we have failed to live up to our own expectations or society's expectations for us.

Our emotions are heavily influenced by our conscience and values. Therefore, our conscience might be responsible for our feelings of guilt, shame, embarrassment, or, conversely, pride.

Our emotions are frequently positive influences in our lives. They may either inspire our creativity or motivate us to accomplish worthy things in the world. Anger, for instance, may motivate us to get out of abusive relationships or to fight injustice in our community and world; boredom may be the impetus for us to begin to make changes in our life; and love for others may inspire us to work more cooperatively with them. Furthermore, as discussed in chapter 5, our passions are a measure of our spirit.

But our emotions have a dark or negative side. They may cause us to overfocus on or obsess about ourselves, such as occurs with depression; or become destructive by permitting us to vent our anger inappropriately, and cause us to damage our relationships.

And our emotions significantly impact our health. The role of emotions in health is most dramatically revealed in situations such as the following:

- Bernard Lown has described his observations during grand rounds. After diagnosing a woman with tricuspid stenosis (TS) (a narrowing of one of the heart valves), he turned and said to surrounding interns and residents, "This woman has TS." The woman, who interpreted this to mean that she had a "terminal situation," became anxious, breathed rapidly, and died shortly thereafter (Cousins, 1983, pp. 14–15).
- Another patient overheard his doctor tell others that he had a "wholesome gallup," a symptom of a failing heart. The patient believed the use of the word wholesome meant that his heart was hardy. Consequently, he recovered and was discharged from the hospital (ibid., pp. 15–16).
- College graduates who were the most pessimistic members of their class when interviewed in 1946 were the least healthy when studied in 1980 (Myers, 1992, p. 117).
- Depression accounts for an estimated 26,000 deaths/year from ischemic heart disease (Voelker, 1996, p. 345) and has been shown to affect survival in people with AIDS (Mayne, Vittinghoff, Chesney, et al., 1996).
- Fear and grief have both been associated with sudden death (see Cousins, 1983, p. 200 [fear]; Parkes, Benjamin, & Fitzgerald, 1969 [grief]). Sudden death has occurred in people who are physically healthy but who have suffered fright (see

Cousins, 1983, p. 200), confronted grave personal danger (ibid.), or experienced the death of close relatives (ibid.). Sudden death has also been observed in physically ill people who panic because they believe their condition may have taken a turn for the worse.

The role of emotions in health is supported by the fact that happy people often appear to be healthier (Weeks & James, 1995) (see the later discussion of negative moods). Nonconformists and eccentrics[1] are also believed to be healthier because they do not feel obligated to follow social norms. They do what they want to do and they are happier than those who feel that they must conform to society's dictates (ibid., p. 16).

The emotions also play substantial roles in somatization disorders and in psychosomatic illness. In somatization disorders, stress results in physical illness (Helman, 1990, p. 233) (see the highlight box, "A Worldwide Perspective about Somatization Disorders").

In psychosomatic illness, however, people's emotional characteristics, often incorporated into their personality types, apparently cause them to become sick with a particular condition or disease. Persons who suffer from migraine headaches often have repressed anger and/or rage; they are typically meticulous, perfectionists, conscientious, intelligent, neat, inflexible, rigid, resentful, guilt-ridden, and compulsive (Lynch, 1985, pp. 221–22). See the highlight box, "Hypertension as a Psychosomatic Condition."

THE RELATIONSHIP BETWEEN PERSONALITY AND HEALTH

Personality Traits: An Introduction

Lord Byron believed that we are all differently organized (Jamison, 1995, p. 210). Because of this "different organization," we may be born with particular personality traits that, as will be discussed later, may affect our health.

Carl Jung believed that we are born with many personality traits (Dossey, 1993, pp. 92–93; see Singer, 1972, p. 184). Jung believed that, first, we are either extroverts or introverts;[2] second, he believed, humans have four other personality differences, which he named *the four functions*. Two of these functions are rational (feeling and thinking) and two nonrational (intuition and sensation) (Dossey, 1993, p. 93).

The Relationship between Personality Traits and Health

In the East, some medical systems are predicated on the belief that health is affected by one's personality type; one example is *Ayurveda*, an Indian medical tradition

A WORLDWIDE PERSPECTIVE ABOUT SOMATIZATION DISORDERS

Toward a Clearer Definition of Somatization

Some have defined *somatization* "as the expression of personal and social distress in an idiom of bodily complaints and medical help seeking" (Kleinman & Kleinman, 1985, p. 430). Patients who somatize *amplify* their bodily symptoms and *minimize* their affective and cognitive problems (ibid., p. 472). A group of American researchers studied 100 Chinese patients diagnosed by Chinese doctors with "neurasthenia," an emotional and psychic disorder characterized by impaired interpersonal relationships and often by fatigue, depression, feelings of inadequacy, headaches, hypersensitivity to sensory stimuli (e.g., light or noise), and psychosomatic symptoms (*Webster's New Collegiate Dictionary*, 1981, p. 765). All the patients diagnosed with neurasthenia believed that their problems were primarily physical—they did not consider themselves depressed—even though they attended a psychiatric clinic (Kleinman & Kleinman, 1985, p. 439).

The Manifestations of Somatization

Stress and depression are just two conditions that cause some individuals to somatize in different cultures (Helman, 1990; Kleinman & Good, 1985). And, as noted, many people with somatization disorders do not consider themselves depressed (Kleinman & Kleinman, 1985, p. 439).

The fact that somatization may manifest disease in different organs has been described as "organ choice" (Helman, 1990, p. 251). For example, Americans experiencing stress tend to report gastrointestinal symptoms; the French experience changes in mood or thought content; and Filipinos emphasize rapid heartbeat and shortness of breath (Guthrie, Verstraete, Deines, et al., 1975). Consider some of the results of studies on somatization and depression:

- Depressed Indonesian patients had loss of vitality and somatic symptoms, whereas Germans reported having decreased efficiency, feelings of guilt, and suicidal tendencies (Pfeiffer, 1968).

- Londoners and Nigerians both reported depressed mood. However, Londoners increasingly reported feelings of guilt, anxiety, and active contemplation of suicide, whereas Nigerians were more likely to experience somatization and motor retardation (Binitie, 1975).

The Prevalence and Distribution of Somatization Disorders throughout the World

Somatization cases account for between one third and three fourths of patient visits to primary care physicians in the United States and United Kingdom (Kleinman & Kleinman, 1985, p. 434). In many cultures, particularly in China, Hong Kong, and Japan, somatization disorders are given particular credence (see Lau, Kung, & Chung, 1983 [Hong Kong]; Tseng, 1975 [China]; Wang, 1983 [China]; Weil, 1995, p. 91 [Japan]). In part, the prevalence of somatization in the East may be explained by the fact that it is considered inappropriate to talk about emotions (see Moyers, 1993, p. 274). The Vietnamese and Chinese, among others, do not feel that it is "legitimate" to discuss the symptoms of depression with doctors—although it is acceptable to discuss such symptoms with family, friends, priests, and even fortune-tellers (Beiser, 1985, p. 286).

The Causes of Somatization

Many personal and social reasons have been suggested to account for the presence of somatization disorders (see Kleinman & Kleinman, 1985). Several have pointed to the strong association between worker dissatisfaction and symptoms: in Chinese patients with somatization disorders (which largely included depression and/or the presence of pain), 43 percent expressed their dislike of their work and 33 percent indicated a strong desire to change their work (ibid., p. 446). Others have concluded that somatization of personal and social distress constitutes a large component of disability payments and missed workdays and is also frequently an emblem of worker dissatisfaction (Alexander, 1982; Yelin, Nevitt, & Epstein, 1980). Other factors that have been considered to mediate a patient's somatization disorder include family and marital problems, economic difficulties, and, among Chinese patients, "political problems" (Kleinman & Kleinman, 1985, p. 452). Consider the "political problems" of one individual, now in his 20s, who suffers from chronic headaches and dizziness and is diagnosed with chronic neurotic depression (ibid., p. 455).

As a 12-year-old boy during the Cultural Revolution, this individual found an anti-Mao slogan ("Throw down Chairman Mao") tacked to the rear door of his school. The boy ran to his close friend who suggested that he take the slogan and bring it to the attention of their Commune leaders. These leaders called the police, who told the boy that if he did not confess he could not return home. Although he told the police he was the person who found the slogan and did not write it, and although he was allowed to return home, the next morning three "agents" came to his home and took him away to be interrogated. Terrified that he would not be allowed to return home, he signed the confession and accepted sole responsibility for writing the poster. He also told his mother that he wrote the poster and she remarked "If I knew before you'd end up like this, I wouldn't have wanted you." Because of his confession, the youth was marched through his town wearing a dunce cap and carrying a sign around his neck in which he had written some self-criticism for his act. The townspeople cursed him, spat at him, and threw dirt and pebbles at him. The next day the youth was sent to work as a peasant at a local commune and perform the work of an adult. After a year of hard labor, the other peasants were able to get the youth re-admitted to school. This patient believes that this incident has affected his character. (ibid., pp. 455–58)

Personality and Other Characteristics of Persons with Somatization Disorders

Apparently psychiatrists and psychologists regard somatization as a "maladaptive coping style" (ibid., p. 474), a means of coping with emotional problems such as discharging anger in a sanctioned way, fulfilling dependency needs, and dealing with perceived failure (ibid.). Others conclude that persons who are at greatest risk for powerlessness and "blocked access to local resources" are most likely to somatize (ibid., p. 475).

Experts have observed that the following groups are prone to somatization: ethnic and refugee populations (ibid.); working-class patients who attend pain clinics for low back pain (ibid.); women, particularly those experiencing chronic pain (ibid.); and Catholics (versus Protestants) (Shweder, 1985, p. 196).

The Treatment of Somatization Disorders

In the study of Chinese patients diagnosed with "neurasthenia," the Chinese psychiatrists who made this diagnosis viewed their patients' problems as biological—even though, according to the American doctors, the Chinese patients all had somatization disorders (Kleinman & Kleinman, 1985, p. 439).

This study might suggest that the traditional Chinese medical system does not treat a patient's emotional "imbalances." The following data, however, may suggest otherwise. According to principles of Traditional Chinese Medicine (TCM), "liver" is a metaphor for anger, "heart" for anxiety, "spleen" for depression, and "kidney" for a decline in reproductive powers (Ots, 1990). Therefore, it is not surprising that in one TCM Clinic in Nanjing, about 80 percent of liver-related diagnoses given did not relate to actual physical disease but to "aspects of anger" (Helman, 1994, p. 270). Treatments in such a clinic, therefore, consist of herbs to treat one's liver and one's "liver-anger."

(see the highlight box). Consider the following data suggesting a strong association between personality traits and health:

- Persons with chronic anxiety, long periods of sadness and pessimism, tension or incessant hostility, relentless cynicism or suspiciousness, have double the risk of diseases such as asthma, headaches, peptic ulcers, and heart disease (Friedman & Booth-Kewley, 1987).
- Persons who consider themselves rational and pride themselves on never showing their anger often have greatly increased rates of heart disease, cancer, and stroke (Grossarth-Maticek, Bastiaans & Kanazir, 1985).
- People with high needs for power, because of the importance they attribute to impressing and influencing others, often have higher blood pressures and are sick more often than those without such power needs (McClelland, 1976).

Although it is not quite clear how emotions contribute to the day-to-day development of illness, scientific studies are beginning to examine the havoc that emotions can cause on cells and tissues. A study linking despair with an increase in the prevalence of atherosclerosis in middle-aged men used ultrasound scans to document the level of narrowing in patients' arteries (Everson, Kaplan, Goldberg, et al., 1997).

Different personality characteristics, partially reflected by different coping styles (see the section, "The Health-Related Implications of Different Coping Styles"), may affect our health. It is well accepted that persons with Type A personality are at increased risk for heart disease. Although others have suggested that there may also be a Type C or cancer-prone personality (Temoshok, 1987), this hypothesis has met much resistance (Hawkins, 1993, p. 140), despite studies that seem to support it. This resistance is due to beliefs that

---

HYPERTENSION AS A PSYCHOSOMATIC CONDITION

Many researchers have stated the belief that hypertensive patients may have experienced psychological conflicts in early childhood (Alexander, French, & Pollock, 1968; Moses, Daniels, & Nickerson, 1956; Lynch, 1985; Reiser, Rosenbaum, & Ferris, 1951; Weiner, 1979). As adults, they often hid their feelings of anger and aggression and appeared friendly, submissive, and unassertive (Lynch, 1985, p. 96). Presumably, they hid their feelings of aggression because they feared losing the affection of others (Alexander, French, & Pollock, 1968, p. 20), particularly of those on whom they depended (Lynch, 1985, p. 96). Therefore, such adult patients often unconsciously demanded to be taken care of.

Prior to the widespread use of antihypertensives in the 1950s, many physicians sought to control patients' hypertension by providing psychotherapy either to enable patients' to develop insight into the source of their problems or to provide emotional support and reassurance (ibid., pp. 94–95). These efforts apparently had mixed results (ibid.).

---

either individuals will blame themselves for having caused their illness or that once the causes of the illness are removed (such as certain personality traits), the course of the illness will be reversed (ibid.). Last, some experts believe that persons with certain personality profiles are more predisposed to certain psychosomatic conditions.

The Type A Personality. Persons with a Type A personality are said to be hostile and to suffer from "hurry sickness" (Friedman & Rosenman, 1974). They speak faster and louder than others, tend to speak over others, and use more emphatic gestures when they talk (Lynch, 1985, p. 141). Many physiological changes have been measured in persons with Type A personalities. For example, although the very act of speaking increases one's blood pressure; the higher patients' resting blood pressure, the more it increases while speaking (ibid., p. 132). Because persons with Type A personalities often speak more quickly and loudly than others, they experience an immediate increase in both blood pressure and heart rate (ibid., p. 145).

The Type C Personality. Although Temoshok was the first to refer to a Type C personality, many researchers, including Temoshok, have described the personality traits of those believed to be at high risk for cancer. They include persons who

- are stoic, nice, industrious, perfectionist, sociable, and conventional (Temoshok, 1987);
- have difficulty expressing emotions (ibid.);
- have a poor outlet for emotional discharge (Kissen, 1964);
- have attitudes that make them resigned or helpless/hopeless (Grossarth-Maticek, Bastiaans, & Kanazir, 1985; Temoshok, 1987);
- are rational and antiemotional (Grossarth-Maticek, Bastiaans, & Kanazir, 1985; Grossarth-Maticek, Siegrist, & Vetter, 1982). One long-term follow-up study of 1,353 persons in Yugoslavia showed that the incidence of cancer was forty times higher in research subjects who answered positively to 10 or 11 questions to assess their rationality/antiemotionality (Grossarth-Maticek, Bastiaans, & Kanazir, 1985).[3]

As already mentioned, there is resistance to the notion that there may be a cancer-prone personality,[4] because of a belief that people will blame themselves for having caused their own illness or might also come to believe that they "deserve" an illness, as a judgment for "having done something wrong" or "evil." It is important to remember that although people who have cancer may have certain personality traits, the development of cancer may be a complex process, including such other factors as poor nutrition; for example, those in the lowest quartile, who consume few fruits and vegetables, have *twice* the rate of cancer for all cancers except breast cancer (Volker, 1995).

There is currently much debate (and usually agreement) in the medical literature that asthma is a psychosomatic condition (Meijer, Griffioen, van Nierop, et al., 1995). The high incidence of asthma among children who live in ghettos (Belluck, 1996)[5] is attributed to "arduous living conditions," including stress at home (ibid.).

The Personality Profile of Someone with Psychosomatic Conditions. There is some controversy in recognizing disease as psychosomatic: in the West few diseases are considered psychosomatic; in the East many diseases are (Weil, 1995, pp. 89–91).[6]

People with psychosomatic illness are frequently diagnosed with alexithymia, an inability to communicate effectively about their emotions (Lynch, 1985, pp. 230–40). *Alexithymia,* meaning "without words for feelings" (ibid., p. 230), was first formally characterized by Dr. Peter Sifneos in the 1970s as a communication disorder typically observed in persons with psychosomatic illness (Sifneos, 1973). Some have suggested that alexithymia may not be a unique disorder but rather "a facet of the better-measured repressive style" (Bonanno & Singer, 1990).

Communication is an "intimate form of sharing" (Lynch, 1985, p. 243). Consequently, to be comfortable communicating with others, one must believe that one's world is worth being invited into (ibid.). If one faces emotional pain, it is difficult to invite others into one's world and engage in "real" talk. In fact, when persons with alexithymia engage in "real" talk, their cardiovascular system responds as if they were terrorized (ibid., p. 244).

In addition to having difficulty sharing their feelings, persons with alexithymia typically

AYURVEDA: AN ANCIENT MEDICAL TRADITION

Ayurveda developed from the ancient books of wisdom known as the *Vedas* (Svoboda, 1996, p. 67). Over the years, it has been influenced by the Greek Hippocratic tradition and the Arabic medical tradition (the Unani) (Desai, 1989, p. 12). Since the Ayurvedic texts place the medical tradition "squarely within the larger province of traditional religious pursuits and philosophy," it is not surprising that the tradition incorporates central concepts of Hinduism (ibid., p. 75). But Ayurveda is also practiced in Sri Lanka (Nordstrom, 1989) and Tibet (Sachs, 1995), and in these cultures the medical tradition incorporates central tenets of Buddhism.

Ayurveda means the "science of life" or "the wisdom of longevity" (ibid.) and embodies the philosophy that people are what they "eat, think, and do" (ibid., p. 77). Ayurveda is a holistic system that considers the relationships among the body, mind, and spirit. Ayurvedic practitioners (or *vaidyas*) evaluate where patients are at the moment, how much and in what direction they are changing, what influences are affecting that change, and what can be done to make their states more harmonious and their "life momentums rhythmic" (Svoboda, 1996, p. 82).

In Ayurveda, the fundamental energy of life is expressed through three *doshas*—the *vada, pitta,* or *kosha* (Dollemore, Giuliucci, Haigh, et al., 1995). When there is an imbalance in the body, the doshas are either overproduced or underproduced, "at the expense of the body's vitality, adaptability and immunity" (Svoboda, 1996, p. 74). In analyzing the body's vitality (or the individual's "personal constitution"), vaidyas assess the body's "digestive fire" and "bowel predisposition" (ibid., p. 76); for example, when the doshas are in balance, stress to the intestines is not likely to cause either diarrhea or constipation (ibid.). Each of these doshas is associated with different personality traits and physical characteristics (Dollemore, Giuliucci, Haigh, et al., 1995). Practitioners must determine which dosha is predominant or secondary in patients. Some patients are treated solely by altering their diet.

Ayurvedic medicine posits a close relationship between people's personalities and the presence of certain medical ailments (see Chopra, 1991; Dollemore, Giuliucci, Haigh, et al., 1995). As a result, vaidyas are likely to prescribe certain foods for persons with specific personality traits.

This ancient system of medicine also recognizes patients' varied abilities to cope with illness. Major diseases may seem minor in people who have "richness of spirit" or who have "strong minds"—those who have "strong memories, devotion, gratitude, wisdom, purity, great energy, skill, courage, freedom from sorrow, firmness of tread, intelligence, character" (ibid.). Conversely, minor diseases may seem major in patients with a "poverty" of those traits (ibid.).

Diagnosis is often based on taking the patient's pulse and inspecting the patient's face and tongue (Desai, 1989, p. 87). Treatments may be quite varied. Patients' diets may be altered (fasting may be recommended), their horoscopes considered (ibid., p. 12), and they may be prescribed roots, leaves, or bark from a vast pharmacopeia (ibid., p. 82). Vaidyas commonly use urines (Svoboda, 1992, p. 92). Mercury is also the most important metal used in Ayurvedic therapies; it is reacted with sulfur to detoxify it (ibid.).

Ayurveda is still practiced in India today. From 1835, and during the following 100 years of British rule in India, however, state patronage of Ayurvedic institutions was "completely cut off" (Shankar & Manohar, 1996, p. 100). In 1971, the Central Council of Indian Medicine was established to bring uniformity and maintain educational standards in Ayurveda. Today, India has 264,800 registered vaidyas and 4769 licensed pharmacies for the manufacture of Ayurvedic medicines (ibid., p. 101).

- discuss matters in a logical and rational way (ibid., p. 238): As a result, they often succeed in professions such as medicine, nursing, engineering, science, psychology, education, and law (ibid., p. 236).
- exhibit sterile or monotonous ideas (Krystal, 1979): As a result, their thoughts are often composed of trivial details of their everyday life and they seem unable to get beyond mundane preoccupations (ibid.).
- have impoverished imaginations, which lead to impaired creativity (ibid.).
- show poor attentiveness to their body and health (ibid.).

TAKING CHARGE OF OUR EMOTIONS

Frequently, our emotions may cause us to focus inward: anger causes us to focus on why we are right and another is wrong, and sadness causes us to focus on our hurts and worries. To the extent that our emotions cause us to focus upon ourselves, they may prevent us from doing what is necessary, and taking the steps needed to accomplish our goals.

One way to subvert the power of our emotions is to employ regular use of meditation—mental discipline that enables us to remain calm and centered. The calming effect of meditation is illustrated by the fact that it can reduce blood pressure by 20 percent (Pelletier, 1977, p. 213). It is also reputed to restore energy to levels greater than those experienced in deep sleep (ibid., pp. 193, 197).

Meditation trains us not to react to every thought that comes into our mind (see Kabat-Zinn, 1990, p. 65). Once we become aware that not every thought that enters our mind is critical, we keep our lives in "perspective." Consequently, meditation's aim has been said to be to allow us to get mastery over our "attention" (Pelletier, 1977, p. 193). One effect of gaining mastery over our attention is a greater sense of control. Meditators are more likely to experience an inner locus of control (ibid., p. 200), although this may be attributed to the fact that they are likely to make many life-style and behavioral changes.

THE IMPACT OF STRESS AND EMOTIONAL
AROUSAL UPON HEALTH

Stress is generally agreed to be the way in which we respond to or perceive particular events. Many have studied the impact of stress upon health. The following events have been found to be stressful and to have an adverse impact on people's health:

- Immigration or moving to a foreign country, in part because immigrants must learn to adapt to a new culture (see Helman, 1990, p. 245).
- Illiteracy and the social isolation associated with it (see Dossey, 1991, pp. 70–71).
- Uncertainty (see Pelletier, 1977, p. 89): As discussed later, our response to uncertainty may be that we cannot exert as much control in our life as we'd like.
- Fathers' anticipation of the birth of their children (Lipkin & Lamb, 1982): Researchers have defined the couvade syndrome as "involving the occurrence of physical/psychological symptoms in the mates of pregnant women, for which they sought medical care and which were not otherwise objectively explained" (ibid.).[7]

Some people do not respond to certain events as stressful, whereas others do (see Antonovsky, 1979; Maddi & Kobasa, 1984). Several mediating variables, such as our coping style or the amount of social support we have, can influence our response to any stressor.

Even events of a positive nature (e.g., marriage, job change) can be stressful and ultimately affect our health (see Holmes & Masuda, 1973). Because Holmes and Masuda observed a strong correlation between the intensity of life changes and the onset of severe illness, they devised a "Social Readjustment Rating Scale," which assigned numerical values to events in people's lives (e.g., divorce, marriage, death in the family). Individuals who scored over 300 points on the scale had a 90 percent likelihood of experiencing health changes.

The Physiological Characteristics of Stress and Control

During arousal, levels of certain chemicals become elevated in our bodies; many, such as cortisol, impair the immune system (Justice, 1987, p. 84). Furthermore, people with high needs for power have chronic activation of the sympathetic nervous system and, therefore, lower levels of immune function (ibid., p. 249). Dopamine level is depleted in the brain if we believe a situation is uncontrollable (ibid., pp. 84, 191)—for example, feeling trapped in a bad job or marriage. Even an "anxiety peptide," a small molecule that apparently increases anxiety, has been discovered in the brain (Marx, 1985).

The Mind's Capacity to Amplify Events

A minute event, thought, or emotion can have significant influence on the body (Pelletier, 1977, p. 34). Consequently, the brain may amplify thoughts about "living" or "dying" and send these messages to the body. As discussed in the section, "The Will to Live and Purpose in Life," it is surprising how quickly people die once they give up hope. Worries and negative expectations may translate into physical illness "because the body feels as if we are endangered, even if the threat is imaginery" (Ferguson, 1980, p. 251).

Once the brain amplifies a thought or emotion, it may take some time for the resulting stimulation to subside. The mind may remain "psychologically stressed" even when the body relaxes; for example, during stress, a person's muscle activity (as measured by an electromyogram) and brain activity (as measured by an electroencephalogram) may increase (Pelletier, 1977, p. 80). But during relaxation, it is common only for the activity indicated by the EMG to decrease—brain activity as measured by the EEG is still increased (ibid.). Meditation, however, enables people to "recover" more quickly from stress-inducing events (ibid., p. 206).

THE NATURE AND VALUE OF THE POSITIVE EMOTIONS

In the 1970s, the term *hardiness* was used to describe psychologic variables that "strengthen a person's ability to resist 'debilitating effects'" (Kobasa, 1979). Hardiness was believed to consist of three components: control, commitment, and challenge (ibid.).

Positive emotions enable us to live life. They enable us to do more than exist and merely react to circumstances as they arise. They allow us to be proactive and do the things that we feel passionate about, that enrich our lives and give them meaning. These positive emotions include the will to live and the ability to experience purpose in life, the ability to establish a sense of control, the capacity to learn to accept one's circumstances (for acceptance is often the springboard toward meaningful growth and development), a positive attitude, and capacity to maintain happiness, hope, and optimism.

The Will to Live and Purpose in Life

He who has a why to live for can bear with almost any how.
Friedrich Nietzsche
quoted in Frankl,
Man's Search for Meaning, p. 121

Goals—heartfelt, passionate goals—are like anchors in deep water. When I get into I-don't-want-to-live thinking, I remind myself I have an anchor out there.
Jay Stinson, diagnosed with AIDS in 1975
quoted in Lederer (with Kathy DeLeon),
"The Newest AIDS Treatment Is Not a Drug," p. 62

Studies of the survivors of the concentration camps have analyzed why some people succumbed in the camps and others survived (Dimsdale, 1974; Frankl, 1963).[8] The survivors focused on the good (Dimsdale, 1974) and their purpose for survival, such as something they had to look forward to, whether it was being reunited with families or finishing meaningful projects (Frankl, 1963, pp. 118–21). As Viktor Frankl has noted, humanity's basic desire is to find meaning in life. This view is distinct from Freud's and Adler's notion that people seek, respectively, pleasure or power.

What seems particularly shocking is that healthy individuals who have apparently lost their will to live often spontaneously get ill and die (ibid.). Frankl, a concentration camp survivor, describes one man in such a camp who had hoped for liberation of his camp by March 30, 1945; actually, the man reported a dream in which he was told that the camp would be liberated on that date (ibid., pp. 118–19). But as this day drew near the war news that reached the camp "made it appear very unlikely that [the camp] would be free[d] on the promised date" (ibid., p. 119). On March 29, this man suddenly became ill with a high temperature. On March 30, he became delirious and lost consciousness, and on March 31, he died (ibid., pp. 119–20). Although Dr. Frankl notes that he apparently died of typhus, he concluded that a latent typhus infection was activated by the man's "loss of hope and courage" (ibid., p. 120).

Dr. Frankl also noted that the chief doctor of his concentration camp informed him that the death rate between Christmas 1944 and New Year's 1945 was the highest it had ever been (ibid., p. 120). The doctor attributed this high death rate to the fact that most "prisoners had lived in [*sic*] the naïve hope that they would be home again for Christmas. As the time drew near and there was no encouraging news, the prisoners lost courage and disappointment overcame them" (ibid., p. 121).

For many people, purpose in life may be attained through work (versus deriving meaning from relationships) (see Storr, 1988, p. 163). Such persons should be reluctant to give up their work completely even as illness-related limitations affect their capacity to be as productive as they once were.

Many people who are independent and nonconformist develop their own sense of meaning and do not necessarily adapt to the norms of their culture. Such persons may seem quite content, if not happy. It may not be surprising, therefore, that, as discussed in chapter 1, nonconformists are usually healthier than conformists (Weeks & James, 1995).

People with chronic and terminal illnesses often attempt to find meaning in their illnesses or suffering (Taylor, 1983)—they ask themselves why they became sick. They also consider the impact of illness on their lives and the meaning of their lives now (ibid., p. 1161). The search for meaning is believed to represent patients' attempts to control their environments.

The Ability to Focus and to Concentrate

We will not be able to experience much meaning or purpose in our lives without the ability to focus and to concentrate. That ability is an important concept in Chinese medicine. The Chinese view health, in part, as the ability to concentrate one's mind upon a particular matter (Moyers, 1993, p. 282). In fact, the distribution of one's energy, or *chi*, is governed by one's will (ibid., p. 310). In other words, what one decides to do governs the distribution of energy in one's body—and according to traditional views of Chinese medicine, all disease results from the inappropriate distribution of energy in the body.

Establishing a Sense of Control

Toward Defining Control. Some have considered control to be

- "a belief that one has at one's disposal a response that can influence the aversiveness of an event" (Justice, 1987, p. 61)
- "the active belief that one has a choice among responses" (Langer, 1983, p. 20)
- "a sense of permanence and continuity" (Boyce, Schaefer, & Uitti, 1985)

Antonovsky's definition of coherence seems almost exclusively to be about maintaining an internal locus of control, the belief that one can shape the nature of one's life. He defines *coherence* as

a global orientation that expresses the extent to which one has a pervasive, enduring though dynamic feeling of confidence that one's internal and external environments are predictable and that there is a high probability that things will work out as well as can be reasonably expected. (Antonovsky, 1979, p. 123)

The concept of control has a significant psychological component, including the ability to decide the type of life one is going to live. As Karl Jaspers said, being human is "deciding what one is going to be" (Frankl, 1975, p. 26). People who believe that they can shape the nature of their lives are said to have an internal locus of control. Psychologists estimate that 20 percent of persons have this belief (Siegel, 1986, p. 167).

Others have defined a sense of control by illustrating that it is not helplessness (as Martin Seligman has defined it) or the belief that one is powerless. Exerting control implies that one is taking responsibility for oneself (see Langer, 1983, p. 101).

Several have postulated a relationship between health and one's perceived sense of control (Engel, 1971; Seeman & Seeman, 1983). Consider some of the following conclusions of studies examining the relationship between health and control:

- In an analysis of 170 cases of sudden death, one researcher attributed it to the subjects' perception that they no longer had any control over their situations (Engel, 1971).
- People with little sense of personal control at work experience greater stress than employees who feel they have a sense of control (Karasek, Russell, & Theorell, 1982) and, as a result, have a substantial and statistically significant elevated risk for mortality from cardiovascular disease (Johnson, Stewart, & Hall, 1996).

Teaching Patients How to Exert Control over Their Health. There are many ways in which patients can exert greater control over their health care:

- Requiring that their physicians give them more information about prescribed drugs (their benefits and side effects) and recommended treatments (prospective outcomes; potential risks).
- Making their own decisions regarding the types of drugs they wish to take for their conditions.
- Asking their doctors more questions: Patients with diabetes who actively conversed with their doctors had lower follow-up glucose levels, a sign of better diabetes control, than patients who did not ask their doctor questions (Kaplan & Greenfield, 1993).
- Using nonmedical means to assist them to reduce their symptoms: Patients with chronic obstructive pulmonary disease can be taught measures to conserve energy; they can also be taught relaxation techniques to reduce their anxiety—because increased anxiety causes greater difficulty in breathing (Narsavage, 1997).

Some patients may wish to make their own health-related decisions and take away a certain amount of control traditionally exerted by doctors. In such situations, the doctor essentially becomes an adviser or facilitator (see Siegel, 1989, p. 125). Dr. Siegel refers to himself as a "facilitator of healing, not a healer." In this model of the doctor/patient relationship, the patient ultimately is the decision maker.

Some doctors will undoubtedly feel uncomfortable with the patient as decision maker. Their egos may not be strong enough to accept patients' disagreement with them about treatment strategy. As already noted, assertive patients who make their own health care decisions may trust their doctors implicitly but may use different objective criteria, for example, to determine whether to initiate particular drug or other therapies.

Certain groups of patients, such as those with AIDS and people with cancer, have initiated a patients rights movement by demanding that they have a large say in their health-related decisions (see Callen, 1990, pp. 195–97; Smith, 1996, pp. 135–37, 141), including their right to take medications that their physicians may feel are either useless or harmful. Patients, particularly as they become more informed about their conditions and the treatments for them, are insisting on making such decisions. Some patients, like Charlotte Streit (see her interview in chapter 2) and Jeff Winograd (see his interview in chapter 8), research the medical literature for different treatment options. Even the interview with Dr. Chris Costas (chapter 2) refers to one patient with AIDS who quite objectively reviewed the data in the medical literature on drugs used to treat HIV-related conditions.

Some patients have underscored the need to remain skeptical about reports on the value or effectiveness of certain therapies (see Callen, 1990, p. 194). Some with AIDS, for example, realize the amount of money pharmaceutical companies can make on AIDS-related drugs and, consequently, may not always believe the advertisements for AIDS-related drugs and treatments. Physicians should not exclusively rely on the information contained in advertisements to determine whether they will prescribe certain drugs; for example, the more physicians rely on "promotion" as their source of information on drugs, the less appropriately they prescribe (Lexchin, 1997). In one study, a panel of experts examined the quality of advertisements for pharmaceutical products in leading medical journals; they found that the advertisements

- often minimized concerns about adverse drug reactions (Wilkes, Doblin, & Shapiro, 1992);
- were misleading with respect to reporting about the efficacy of drugs (ibid.);
- used statistics inappropriately (ibid.); and
- promoted the use of products for "inappropriate patient populations" (ibid.).

THE HEALTH-RELATED IMPLICATIONS
OF DIFFERENT COPING STYLES

Patients with diseases often show a wide array of coping styles that may enable them to adjust to the impact of a disease or to resist acknowledging that they have a disease that exerts an impact upon their life. These coping styles may predict not only patients' quality of life but also their likelihood of survival (see Rodin & Salovey, 1989).

Coping styles, however, may vary from culture to culture. Some cultures take a dim view of the excessive expression of feelings. The Chinese believe that such expression will disturb the body's harmony and lead to illness (Kleinman, 1980). In Bali, active denial of some problems is supported by the culture because "not to think about something" is "not to feel it" (Pennebaker, 1995a, p. 19).

Some physicians have discussed the fact that coping styles may even be affected by how patients have viewed their lives or what their experiences were like (Cassell, 1982, p. 642). Cassell notes that "[i]f cancer occurs in a patient with self-confidence from past achievements, it may give rise to optimism and a resurgence of strength. Even if it is fatal, the disease may not produce the destruction of the person but, rather, reaffirm his or her indomitability. The outcome would be different in a person for whom life had been a series of failures" (ibid.).

Coping styles typically include denial, disclosing of one's feelings (which may include being angry), withholding or repressing of feelings (also called "emotional suppression"), and acceptance. Some experts, however, dispute whether the emotions can be consciously manipulated by being suppressed or repressed (Wegner, Shortt, Blake, et al., 1990, p. 415).

Denial

Denial is a natural psychological defense mechanism that allows people to postpone facing facts or psychologically threatening circumstances. These facts or circumstances can be psychologically threatening because they may require patients to make significant changes and/or adjustments in their lives.

Consider some forms of denial in people at risk for HIV/AIDS:

- In one study, 26 percent of individuals who had engaged in high-risk behavior and had agreed to give blood for an HIV test failed to ask for the test result (McCusker, Stoddard, Mayer, et al., 1988).
- In another study, only 7 percent of sexual and needle-sharing partners of HIV-positive subjects were notified by the subject of their HIV status (Landis, Schoenbach, Weber, et al., 1992).

Though these findings may be shocking, one must remember the many factors that fuel denial in HIV/AIDS patients (see Smith, 1995). These include fear of many types of discrimination (e.g., insurance, housing, employment); fear of abandonment by spouses, children, family members, and friends; fear of ostracism and isolation; and even fears surrounding one's own mortality.

HIV-positive people also fear that various state-related "powers" will be used against them. For instance, HIV-positive mothers sometimes fear that their children will be taken from them, because their intravenous drug usage is considered to render them "unfit" (Ports, 1988), and HIV-positive immigrants fear being deported. When state laws have required mandatory reporting to state officials of the name and address of those who are HIV-positive, there have been substantial decreases in those persons seeking HIV testing within that state (Landis, Schoenbach, Weber, et al., 1992).

Most people who deny that they have an illness delay seeking medical attention and, consequently, treatment. People who worry about having cancer delay seeking help (Helman, 1994, p. 134); as already noted, persons who fear that they may be HIV-positive often refuse to have an HIV test. In 1991, the Centers for Disease Control and Prevention estimated that only 12 percent of people who were HIV-infected knew their serostatus (*America Living with AIDS*, 1991, p. 74), but certainly the remaining 88 percent of individuals who did not know—or did not want to know—their HIV status should have known whether they engaged in behavior that put them at risk for acquiring HIV.

Repressing One's Feelings and Emotions

The biopsychosocial literature is replete with references to the personality characteristics of those known as "repressors" or those having an "avoidant personality" (Singer & Sincoff, 1990, p. 487). Some of their personality traits are summarized in Chart 4-2. Most of the time, repression is believed to have adverse consequences for health.[9] In one study of women with breast cancer, emotional repressors had rates of remission 45 percent lower than those who did not repress their emotions (Schwartz, 1990). The physiological mechanisms by which repression jeopardizes health is unknown. One hypothesis, the opiate-peptide hypothesis, states that repressive coping increases the level of endorphins in the brain, thus causing decreased immune function and hyperglycemia (ibid., pp. 422–23).

Disclosing One's Feelings and Emotions

Many researchers theorize that disclosing feelings and emotions can only have a positive impact on health (see Pennebaker, 1995b, p. 4). Patients with breast cancer who express their anger have a better chance for survival than patients who do not express it (Rodin & Salovey, 1989). This view is supported by studies showing that repression of emotions not only activates the sympathetic division of the autonomic nervous system but suppresses some aspects of the immune system (Gross & Levinson, 1993). Patients with malignant myeloma who expressed their feelings were found to have more immune activity at the site of their lesions than patients who did not do so (see Moyers, 1993, p. 332).

Disclosing one's feelings is a form of catharsis, which has been a common healing practice in many cultures (ibid., p. 191). There are psychological reasons for its healing powers. Sick people who can share their fear, pain, sorrow, and

Chart 4-2
Personality Traits of Repressors

Attribute control of their destinies to powerful others and to chance (Spring & Khanna, 1982)

Are less willing to disclose personal information and viewpoints (Miller & Neussle, 1978)

Emphasize the importance of their rational and non-emotional approach to life (Weinberger, Schwartz, & Davidson, 1979)

Do not generally describe themselves as light-hearted or spontaneous

Often define themselves as individuals who do not become upset

Often avoid potential threats (Weinberger, 1990, p. 374)

May delay seeking appropriate medical treatment (ibid.)

Have identifiable deficits related to self-assertion, empathy, and accurate perception of their own/others' beliefs (ibid.)

Shy away from deep interpersonal involvement (Pellegrine, 1971)

Engage in significantly more individual sports and hobbies (Schwartz, 1990)

anger create room to experience "lightness and joy" (ibid., pp. 332–34). These types of emotions are frequently processed in support groups for people attempting to heal. And, as already mentioned, women with metastatic breast cancer who attended support groups lived twice as long as women who only received standard medical care (Spiegel, Bloom, Kraemer, et al., 1989). In the end, psychological support that allows people to process their feelings may enable them to explore who they are, give them the courage to do what they have always wanted to do, and help them to develop peace of mind amid the crisis.

Accepting One's Situation and Condition

The power of acceptance to foster noteworthy healing, either physically or psychologically, has been underscored by many experts (Dossey, 1993, pp. 31,

64). Acceptance, for one thing, is associated with "better adjustment" to cancer (Carver, Pozo, Harris, et al., 1993).

Whether sick or healthy, we need to learn to accept what we cannot control (see Wakefield, 1995, p. 65) before we can really proceed to live our lives. As the serenity prayer cautions, it takes wisdom to know (and accept) the situations we can control and those we cannot. When we reach this acceptance we can move on with our lives because

- we will be more realistic about the limitations our illnesses have imposed upon us (see Price, 1994, p. 182);
- we will understand the implication that our time on this planet is limited; as a result, we will more likely use time more effectively by prioritizing our goals.

The ability to accept one's situation or condition is also considered to promote healing. As mentioned in chapter 3, accepting a serious or terminal condition is not the same as being resigned to die but implies being at peace with oneself (as opposed to being desperate or frenzied about one's condition), facing the truth, and making the most of the precious moments that may remain in our lives.

Sometimes acceptance is related to spiritual or religious factors. Yujiro Ikemi, who has documented spontaneous regression from cancer, has noted that his patients do not

- lapse into depression, despair, lack of motivation, and fear of death after diagnosis;
- through prayer, ask God to "change their diagnosis" or cure them; and
- accept their cancer diagnosis as a death sentence. They may have an attitude of "renewed commitment and gratitude to God, combined with the belief that God's will was being done, no matter what happened" (Dossey, 1993, pp. 30–31).

Brendan O'Regan, vice president of research for the Institute of Noetic Sciences, has made similar observations (ibid., p. 64).

Acceptance can also be related to psychological factors, including coming to terms with who you really are. Acceptance for persons with HIV/AIDS includes acceptance of not only their HIV status but also their status as gay men or lesbians and/or as intravenous drug users. AIDS progressed more rapidly in HIV-positive men who remained closeted about their homosexuality (Cole, Kemeny, Taylor, et al., 1996, p. 63). Furthermore, secrecy about one's HIV status was also associated with a predicted faster progression of the disease (ibid.).

Having a Positive Attitude and Maintaining Happiness and Optimism

[A good attitude] is the capacity to continue to anticipate future good times and to believe that your life is worth living, that your survival has meaning to yourself or others, that there are still things left for you to learn emotionally, intellectually, and spiritually. [It is] the conviction that you have value, that you matter, that your life is worthwhile and is worth struggling to preserve.

Judith Rabkin, Robert Remien, and Christopher Wilson,
Good Doctors, Good Patients, p. 28

TO MY PATIENTS:
In any illness we both have work to do. [Let me describe your job.] The more serious the illness, the more important it is for you to fight back. You've got to mobilize all your resources—spiritual, emotional, intellectual, physical. Your heaviest artillery will be your will to live.

. . .

Illness is not a laughing matter. . . . Your hopes are my secret weapon. They are the hidden ingredient in any prescription I might write. So I will do everything I can to generate and encourage your confidence in yourself and in the certainty of recovery.

. . .

Sincerely yours,
Your Doctor

Norman Cousins,
Head First, pp. 313–14

The contribution of positive mental outlook to survival has been noted by several authors (Green & Green, 1975; Peterson, Maier, & Seligman, 1993). In one study, 122 men who survived their first heart attack were evaluated for optimism and pessimism (Peterson, Maier, & Seligman, 1993). Eight years later, 21 of the 25 most pessimistic men had died and only 6 of the 25 most optimistic men had died (ibid.). In this study, a positive mental outlook was a better predictor of survival than any medical risk factor (ibid.). Possessing a positive and hopeful attitude has been observed as the only common factor among cancer patients whose cancers went into remission (Green & Green, 1975).

People's subjective attitudes about their health are known often to be more important in predicting their mortality than objective data about their health (Idler, 1992). As discussed in chapter 2, those who say their health is poor are seven times more likely to die than those who describe it as excellent (Dossey, 1991, p. 16). Consequently, persons may be quite sick, but they may seem to do well because they believe they are doing well.

Having a good attitude is related to the amount of hope a person may have. People who are without hope have higher disease and mortality rates (Voelker, 1996). One can continue to have hope even in the wake of diagnosis of a terminal disease. Long-term survivors of AIDS continued to set goals despite their belief that they would not be cured (Rabkin, Remien, Katoff, et al., 1993).

The association between happiness and health (see Okun, Stock, Haring, et al., 1994) is probably most dramatically shown in studies of longevity and in studies of job satisfaction. People who retain a sense of happiness, even if old and in poor health, live longer (Wolf, 1959). This sense of happiness (or contentment) may be associated with the fact that such people have a sense of meaning in their life. It has been noted that the elderly experience deterioration of their health when they have nothing to live for (Justice, 1987, p. 238).

Job dissatisfaction is the best predictor of heart disease, regardless of presence of risk factors for heart disease like elevated cholesterol level or high blood pressure (Dossey, 1991, p. 63; Sales & House, 1971). The second best predictor of surviving heart disease in the study mentioned was "overall happiness" (Sales & House, 1971).[10]

Experiencing Love and Intimacy

Persons who experience love and intimacy in their lives are believed to be healthier than those who do not. The following scientific studies provide the physiologic basis for such beliefs:

- People with high scores on tests measuring intimacy have higher levels of immunoglobulin A (IgA) antibodies and less serious illness (Justice, 1987, p. 257).
- People in love have less lactic acid in their blood—making them less tired—and a higher level of endorphins—making them euphoric (Siegel, 1986, pp. 182–83).
- Rabbits who were fed a high-fat diet but who were shown "love" by being taken out of their cages and petted did not have the hyperlipidemia exhibited by the control group who were not taken out of their cages and petted. The study concluded that love can change the way nutrients are metabolized (Chopra, 1996).
- Psychologists at the University of Miami have studied two groups of premature babies. In one group, infants received gentle, loving stroking for 45 minutes each day. The other group did not receive this extra attention. Babies who were touched daily gained weight and developed so rapidly that they were ready to leave the hospital six days earlier than babies in the control group (see Clinton, 1996, p. 88).
- Dogs, when alone, may have heart rates of 120–160 beats/minute. When a human enters a room and then pets them for two to three minutes, their heart rates can drop to as low as 20–30 beats/minute (Lynch, 1977, p. 168).[11]
- The menstrual cycle of humans is influenced by friendships with other women (McClintock, 1971).

Early studies in animals and children demonstrated the importance of love and showed that its absence affected mortality rate (Montagu, 1970, pp. 200 et seq.). In the early 1920s, Dr. Hammett, who studied rats whose parathyroid glands[12] had been removed, reported a significant difference in mortality rate between rats who had been "gentled and petted" and those whose only contact with humans was incident to routine feeding and cage cleaning (see Hammett, 1921; Hammett, 1922). Although the parathyroid glands had been removed in both groups of rats, Hammett concluded that "the stability of the nervous system induced in rats by gentling and petting produces in them a marked resistance to the loss of the parathyroid secretion which in excitable rats usually results in death from acute parathyroidemia in less than 48 hours" (ibid., 1922).

Several early studies also explained a relationship between love and mortality rate in infants and children. In 1915, Dr. Henry Chapin observed that babies from the "best" homes often suffered from mirasmus because their environments lacked "generously supplied mother love" (Chapin, 1915). Some stunning statistics from studies conducted by René Spitz reported on mortality rates of children raised in nurseries (where infants were looked after by their own mothers) versus those raised in a "Foundlinghome" (an institution where children were raised from their third month by overworked personnel) (Montagu, 1970, p. 208; Spitz, 1949). During the first five years of observation of 239 children, the nursery did not lose a single child through death; however, 37 percent of children in the Foundlinghome died during a two-year observation period (ibid.).[13] This mortality rate was attributed to a lack of emotional interchange between child and mother.

THE NATURE OF NEGATIVE EMOTIONS AND THEIR ADVERSE IMPACT ON HEALTH

Negative emotions, such as anger, depression, despair (associated with loneliness or the death of a loved one), and frustration, often have a substantial and adverse impact upon health.

The Impact of Depression and Despair upon Health

Several studies indicate a strong association between mortality from certain diseases and depression (Anda, Williamson, Jones, et al., 1993 [ischemic heart disease]; Burton, Kline, Lindsay, et al., 1986 [chronic renal failure]; Mayne, Vittinghoff, Chesney, et al., 1996 [AIDS]; McGee, Williams, & Elwood, 1994 [cancer]). As noted earlier, depression associated with ischemic heart disease accounts for an estimated 26,000 deaths per year (Anda, Williamson, Jones, et al., 1993).

Depression is known to induce many physiological changes that adversely affect the cardiovascular and immune systems. It is known to increase the blood pressure and heart rate (Leigh & Reiser, 1980, p. 105). Since 1964, it has been known that cortisol level is elevated in depression but becomes normal when the depression ends (Gibbons, 1964). As already discussed, cortisol damages the immune system.

Depression is also known to produce changes at the cellular level. After exposure to cancer-causing agents, depressed persons have been found to have significantly poorer repair of damaged deoxyribonucleic acid (DNA), a common precursor of the development of cancer (Kiecolt-Glaser & Glaser, 1987). As a result, it is not surprising that some researchers have concluded that depression is more likely to be the cause of cancer than the effect (Shekelle, Raynor, Ostfeld, et al., 1981).

Despair is also an emotion that exerts an adverse impact upon health. Despair might be experienced with the loss of a beloved, frequently a spouse; the loss of one's health; or the feeling of being trapped in a job (Dossey, 1991, p. 61). As the interview with Dennis Watlington at the end of this chapter indicates, despair also includes "feeling trapped in life"—where one has lost the ability to hope, dream, and foresee a future.

The loss of a beloved, for example, has been associated with significant dysfunction of the immune system (see Schleifer, Keller, Camerino, et al., 1983). In one study, although recent widowers had normal numbers of T and beta-lymphocytes, these cells stopped functioning. The normal functioning of these cells could not be stimulated in the test tube by chemicals known to be able to "turn them on" (ibid.). Furthermore, the fact that more fatal heart attacks occur on Monday than on any other day of the week (Rabkin, Mathewson, & Tate, 1980) is attributable to the dread people who hate their jobs feel when facing the beginning of the work week.[14]

The Impact of Isolation and Loneliness upon Health

The evidence that isolation and loneliness adversely impact our health is suggested by the following statistics:

- Unmarried persons, the divorced, and the widowed experience a death rate from heart disease two to five times that of persons who are married (Lynch, 1977, p. 35);
- They also consistently experience higher mortality rates for all causes of death (ibid., p. 38).[15]

CHAPTER SUMMARY

Our emotions are heavily influenced by our conscience and values and frequently motivate us to do either good or evil. They interact with our intellect in important ways. And our emotions significantly affect our health, from playing a substantial role in the development of psychosomatic illness to causing somatization disorders.

Persons with particular personality characteristics often have certain diseases. Persons with a Type A personality have an increased risk for heart disease. The person with a Type A personality is said to suffer from "hurry sickness" and typically speaks faster and louder than others, speaks over others, and uses more emphatic gestures when talking. Although many researchers believe particular personality characteristics lead to the development of cancer and propose the existence of a Type C personality, other researchers deride this concept because it may lead patients to feel guilty for causing their illnesses.

There are many positive emotions that favorably impact our health. These include the will to live and the ability to experience purpose in life, the ability to establish a sense of control, the ability to learn to accept one's circumstances, the existence of a positive attitude, and the maintenance of happiness, hope, and optimism. The will to live is often bolstered when individuals have a purpose for living: whether that purpose is to be reunited with family members or to finish meaningful projects. Dr. Viktor Frankl has given dramatic evidence of concentration camp victims who died suddenly after giving up hope that their concentration camps would be liberated by the Allies.

Persons who maintain a sense of control over their health-related decisions have also been found to have better health than persons who are not active participants in their health care. Some researchers have attributed sudden death to subjects' perceptions that they no longer have any control over their situation. Patients can take more control over their health care by asking their doctors more questions and being more involved in decisions about taking particular drugs or undergoing particular treatments. In fact, diabetics who asked their doctors questions had better control of their diabetes than patients who did not ask questions.

Patients have many coping styles—ranging from denial to acceptance of their conditions. Different coping styles are associated with particular health outcomes, as in the situation of women with metastatic breast cancer in support groups (and beyond the stage of denial) who lived twice as long as women who did not attend such groups and who received only standard medical treatment.

The presence of a positive mental outlook is also associated with survival. A positive and hopeful attitude has been the only common factor observed among cancer patients whose cancers went into remission. And optimistic men who were followed for eight years after their first heart attacks had a better survival rate than pessimistic men.

The effect of love and intimacy on survival has also been demonstrated, largely in studies that show the beneficial effects of support. Love and intimacy may even cause physiological changes such as increasing levels of certain antibodies and endorphins, the latter of which may cause euphoria; decreasing blood levels of lactic acid and, consequently, decreasing fatigue; and changing the metabolism of lipids, which would affect the development of heart disease.

Negative emotions, including depression and despair, also have a profound effect on morbidity and mortality. Depression is associated with 26,000 deaths per year from ischemic heart disease and is also associated with death from chronic renal failure, AIDS, and cancer. Sudden death after the death of a spouse is often attributed to despair and, quite possibly loneliness. The isolation that unmarried persons, the divorced, and the widowed experience may explain why their death rate from heart disease is two to five times that of persons who are married.

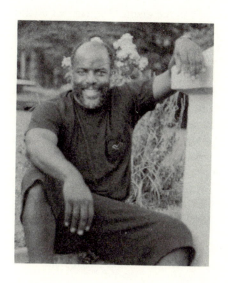

AN INTERVIEW WITH DENNIS WATLINGTON

I am a 45 year old Emmy award–winning filmmaker and live in rural Massachusetts. I was born in Harlem and have been addicted to both heroin and crack. For example, I became a heroin addict when I was 13 1/2 years old and remained a heroin addict until age 16 when I got hepatitis. And I became addicted to crack for about two years when I was aged 32–34. During the periods in which I was an addict, I was also a dealer, because I needed money to support my habit. I was also an alcoholic.

I was able to overcome my addictions through the help of 12-step programs. I attended these programs for about five years. The effectiveness of these programs is due to the nonjudgmental love participants receive; the feeling that participants are not alone and that others are eager to help you even if it is 3 A.M. The 12-step programs also emphasize that while addicts may not be fully responsible for their addictions, they must be accountable to others for the "damage" they have caused. Therefore, the 12-step programs require that addicts make amends for their past behavior and these amends are demonstrated with current changed behavior.

I believe that some of the treatments designed to help the addict, such as methadone maintenance, promote the interests of society but are harmful for the addict. People receiving methadone do not commit crimes, but many have been turned into "zombies." Such "treatments" keep the addict addicted and do not intervene to end the addiction.

Forty percent of my closest friends growing up are deceased. They died from drug overdoses, gang violence and police brutality. Currently, I see a great deal of despair and hopelessness amidst youth living in the ghetto. I remember a term being used by ghetto youth when I grew up in Harlem: "Death is always easier." Today, many youth cannot envision living beyond age 30 and, therefore, they have no hope for the future. In fact, in talking with minority youth at Rikers Island, I was struck by the perception that the "future" for these prisoners may be having lunch. They have lost the courage to hope and dream. I have asked such youth, who has the courage to live to be 30 years old?

At the same time, I believe that experiencing tragedy gives us depth. We must find our own happiness—our society is not obliged to make us happy even though we may be wonderful persons.

Health care for most poor minorities does not provide any informed consent because health professionals do not make the poor aware of their choices. And because the poor may not know that they should have choices (or that they are entitled to them), they are certainly victimized by the health care and medical establishments.

Because blacks have been let down and victimized by authorities, such as by the police, they tend to distrust all authority figures, including doctors and other health care professionals.

I resent the mentality in Western medicine that there must be a prescription for every illness or condition. I would prefer to see more conditions treated without drugs—and possibly with less toxic herbs. I have not been to a traditional Western-trained doctor in many years.

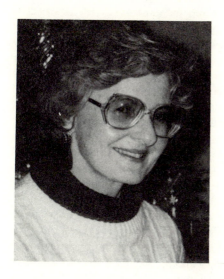

AN INTERVIEW WITH MARY FLYNN WILSON

I'm 59 years old. I was born and brought up in New York City and part of my background is Irish Catholic. I teach English as a second language at a local community college in the Northeast and have been an award-winning journalist and newspaper editor.

I have always been serious and have had to make a conscious effort to have fun. As a teenager, when our family began dating and partying, I felt obligated to watch out for them, to keep them safe and out of trouble. My outlook was pessimistic—I tended to see the glass as half-empty rather than half-full. Many self-help books allowed me to see the glass as half-full. Nevertheless, I used to dread getting up in the morning. I also felt guilty about things that I've done wrong, or imagined that I'd done, including some things that obviously were outside my control. I don't mean to imply that I had no sense of humor, but I often felt burdened and heavy.

Two significant events in my life which have assisted me turn around my perceptions about myself were my diagnosis with a melanoma in 1991 and my mentioning my depression to my treating physician in 1997, who prescribed Prozac to treat it. After my diagnosis with cancer, I read several books by Bernie Siegel. As a result of my reading and being more conscious of my mortality, and the fact that time is limited, I started to take time for myself (and do some of the things I wanted to do); I also learned to "be myself" or more comfortable with who I am.

For a little over a year, I have been on the anti-depressant Prozac. It was not until I began to wake up happily each morning and be thankful for each new day, that I became aware that I had been depressed for most of my life. I felt as if there were a person inside me—a happy person—who had never before been able to get out. Although many members of my immediate family have actually been hospitalized for clinical depression, until November 1997, no doctor ever discussed depression with me, so it has never been officially diagnosed. But in 1997, after filling out a medical questionnaire at my treating physician's office, I answered many questions about my physical condition and emotional feelings. After I admitted to being depressed, my doctor discussed depression with me. Within a few weeks of being put on a low dose of Prozac, I noticed a dramatic improvement in my mood: I felt happy upon waking up and most mornings I started to sing. I also noted a change in my personality—I not only started to stick up for myself, rather than let others "walk all over me," but I became more confident; always fearful of speaking in public, I suddenly found myself giving a long and well-received presentation at a conference and have continued to be able to make public presentations—a bit nervous at the beginning, sometimes, but not paralyzed with terror. In the past, I managed to get through a series of difficult events, including a divorce and working two jobs to put my three children through college on my own, and I thought I had escaped the family history of depression. Somewhere, at some time, some medical professional should have noticed, or routinely inquired about, my depression or at least my family's emotional background.

I am aware of the stigma associated with mental conditions. My grandmother, with whom I lived until I was 20, twice attempted suicide and was confined to a psychiatric hospital for years. We children were never told, partially because of the prevailing attitudes about suicide and emotional illness. But perhaps also because before calling a doctor, my family called a priest, who counseled them not to talk about the incident again. I have heard people of various faiths comment that if people had enough faith, they would be able to overcome mental and emotional problems; suicide was, of course, an even greater assault on these beliefs.

NOTES

1. According to the authors, five traits that apply to virtually every eccentric are nonconforming, creative, strongly motivated by curiosity, idealistic (meaning a desire to make the world a better place and the people in it happier), and happily obsessed with usually five to six "hobbyhorses" (Weeks & James, 1995, pp. 27–28).

2. These beliefs are consistent with more recent studies that suggest that shyness is inherited (Goleman, 1995, pp. 215–16). Some believe that there are four temperamental types that are established at birth: timid, bold, upbeat, and melancholy (ibid.).

3. The questions about personality included the following: If someone deeply hurts your feelings, do you nevertheless try to treat him rationally and to understand his way of behaving? Do you try to understand others even if you do not like them? Does your rationality prevent you from attacking others, even if there are sufficient reasons for doing so?

4. An association between personality type and cancer does not establish a causal connection.

5. As many as 10–20 percent of schoolchildren in Brooklyn suffer from some of the symptoms of asthma (Belluck, 1996).

6. Weil believes that only bronchial asthma and rheumatoid arthritis are psychosomatic (Weil, 1995, pp. 89–90). Since the 1960s, he has also thought that peptic ulcer and ulcerative colitis could be psychosomatic.

7. In their study, these authors reported that 225 of 1000 men were affected by couvade syndrome.

8. What is amazing about those who found themselves in concentration camps is that relatively few people committed suicide by running into the electrified wire surrounding many camps.

9. One notable exception is for those individuals who, immediately after a heart attack, remain in denial and, consequently, remain calm. For example, coronary patients who were admitted to hospitals because they suffered from angina or a heart attack and who did not give in to anxiety and alarm encountered fewer medical problems (including those that were fatal) during the critical first few days, than those who were highly fearful (Gentry & Williams, 1975).

10. The correlation coefficient supporting this association was .83.

11. In some cases, the heart rate slows to such an extent that sinus arrest occurs and the heart pauses for six to eight seconds (Lynch, 1977, p. 168).

12. The parathyroid glands function to maintain normal calcium balance in the body. They comprise four small endocrine glands adjacent to or embedded in the thyroid gland (Webster's Third New International Dictionary, 1971, p. 1640).

13. This study also showed a significant decline in the development quotient (DQ) (a measure of a child's perception, use of body functions, social relations, memory and imitation, manipulative ability, and intelligence) between children raised in the nursery and those raised in the Foundlinghome, even though the children raised in the Foundlinghome had a higher DQ at the beginning of the study (Montagu, 1970, p. 208).

14. Most heart attacks apparently occur at 9:00 A.M. (Muller, Ludmer, Willich, et al., 1987).

15. Although this is United States–based information, the same findings are apparently also true in Japan (Lynch, 1977, p. 48).

SUGGESTED READINGS

Frankl, Viktor. *Man's Search for Meaning: An Introduction to Logotherapy.* Boston:
    Beacon Press, 1962.
Justice, Blair. *Who Gets Sick: Thinking and Health.* Houston: Peak Press, 1987.
Moyers, Bill. *Healing and the Mind.* New York: Doubleday, 1993.

REFERENCES

Alexander, Franz, Thomas M. French, and George H. Pollock. *Psychosomatic Specificity.*
    Chicago: University of Chicago Press, 1968.
Alexander, L. "Illness Maintenance and the New American Sick Role." In *Clinically
    Applied Anthropology.* N. Chrisman and T. Maretzki, eds. Dordrecht: D. Reidel,
    1982, pp. 351–68.
America Living with AIDS: Transforming Anger, Fear and Indifference into Action.
    Report of the National Commission on Acquired Immunodeficiency Syndrome,
    1991.
Anda, R., D. Williamson, D. Jones, et al. "Depressed Affect, Hopelessness, and the Risk
    of Ischemic Heart Disease in a Cohort of U.S. Adults." 4 *Epidemiology* 285–94
    (1993).
Antonovsky, Aaron. *Health, Stress and Coping.* San Francisco: Jossey-Bass, 1979.
Beiser, Morton. "A Study of Depression among Traditional Africans, Urban North
    Americans, and Southeast Asian Refugees." In *Culture and Depression: Studies in
    the Anthropology and Cross-Cultural Psychiatry of Affect and Disorder.* A.
    Kleinman and B. Good, eds. Berkeley: University of California Press, 1985, pp.
    272–98.
Belluck, Pam. "With Asthma Rising, Expanded Health Sessions for Pupils and Parents."
    N.Y. Times, Sept. 29, 1996, p. 39.
Binitie, Ayo. "A Factor-Analytical Study of Depression Across Cultures (African and
    European)." 127 *British Journal of Psychiatry* 559–63 (1975).
Bonanno, George A., and Jerome L. Singer. "Repressive Personality Style: Theoretical
    and Methodological Implications for Health and Pathology." In *Repression and
    Dissociation: Implications for Personality Theory, Psychopathology and Health.*
    J.L. Singer, ed. Chicago: University of Chicago Press, 1990, pp. 435–70.
Boyce, W. Thomas, Catherine Schaefer, and Chris Uitti. "Permanence and Change:
    Psychological Factors in the Outcome of Adolescent Pregnancy." 21 *Social Science
    and Medicine* 1279–87 (1985).
Burton, Howard J., Stephen A. Kline, Robert M. Lindsay, et al. "The Relationship of
    Depression to Survival in Chronic Renal Failure." 48 *Psychosomatic Medicine* 261–
    69 (March/April 1986).
Callen, Michael. *Surviving AIDS.* New York: HarperCollins, 1990.
Carver, Charles S., Christina Pozo, Suzanne D. Harris, et al. "How Coping Mediates the
    Effects of Optimism on Distress: A Study of Women with Early Stage Breast
    Cancer." 65 *Journal of Personality and Social Psychology* 375–90 (Aug. 1993).
Cassell, Eric. "The Nature of Suffering and the Goals of Medicine." 306 *New England
    Journal of Medicine* 639–45 (1982).
Chapin, Henry D. "A Plea for Accurate Statistics in Infants' Institutions." 27
    Transactions of the American Pediatric Society 180 (1915).
Chopra, Deepak. *Perfect Health: The Complete Mind/Body Guide.* New York: Harmony

Books, 1991.

―――. Television lecture on Connecticut Public Television, 1996.

Clinton, Hillary Rodham. *It Takes a Village: And Other Lessons Children Teach Us.* New York: Simon & Schuster, 1996.

Cole, Steve W., Margaret E. Kemeny, Shelley E. Taylor, et al. "Accelerated Course of Human Immunodeficiency Virus Infection in Gay Men Who Conceal Their Homosexual Identity." 58 *Psychosomatic Medicine* 219–31 (May 1996).

Cousins, Norman. *Head First: The Biology of Hope.* New York: E.P. Dutton, 1989.

―――. *The Healing Heart: Antidotes to Panic and Helplessness.* New York: W. W. Norton, 1983.

Desai, Prakash N. *Health and Medicine in the Hindu Tradition: Continuity and Cohesion.* New York: Crossroad, 1989.

Dimsdale, Joel E. "The Coping Behavior of Nazi Concentration Camp Survivors." 131 *American Journal of Psychiatry* 792–97 (1974).

Dollemore, Doug, Mark Giuliucci, Jennifer Haigh, et al. *New Choices in Natural Healing.* B. Gottlieb, S.G. Berg, and P. Fisher, eds. Emmaus, PA: Rodale Press, 1995.

Dossey, Larry. *Meaning and Medicine: A Doctor's Tales of Breakthrough and Healing.* New York: Bantam, 1991.

―――. *The Power of Prayer and the Practice of Medicine.* San Francisco: HarperSan Francisco, 1993.

Engel, George L. "Sudden and Rapid Death During Psychological Stress: Folklore or Folk Wisdom?" 74 *Annals of Internal Medicine* 771–82 (1971).

Everson, Susan A., George A. Kaplan, Debbie E. Goldberg, et al. "Hopelessness and 4-Year Progression of Carotid Atherosclerosis: The Kuopio Ischemic Heart Disease Risk Factor Study." 17 *Arteriosclerosis, Thrombosis and Vascular Biology* 1490–95 (Aug. 1997).

Ferguson, Marilyn. *The Aquarian Conspiracy: Personal and Social Transformation in Our Time.* New York: G.P. Putnam, 1980.

Frankl, Viktor E. *Man's Search for Meaning: An Introduction to Logotherapy.* New York: Pocket Books, 1963.

―――. *The Unconscious God: Psychotherapy and Theology.* New York: Simon & Schuster, 1975.

Friedman, Howard S., and Stephanie Booth-Kewley. "The Disease-Prone Personality: A Meta-Analytic View of the Construct." 42 *American Psychologist* 539–55 (June 1987).

Friedman, Meyer, and Ray H. Rosenman. *Type A Behavior and Your Heart.* New York: Knopf, 1974.

Gentry, W.D., and R.B. Williams. *Psychosocial Aspects of Myocardial Infarction and Coronary Care.* St. Louis: C.V. Mosby, 1975.

Gibbons, James L. "Cortisol Secretion Rate in Depressive Illness." 10 *Archives of General Psychiatry* 572–75 (June 1964).

Goleman, Daniel. *Emotional Intelligence.* New York: Bantam, 1995.

Green, Elmer, and Alyce Green. *Beyond Biofeedback.* New York: Delta, 1975.

Gross, James J., and Robert W. Levinson. "Emotional Suppression: Physiology, Self-Report, and Expressive Behavior." 64 *Journal of Personality and Social Psychology* 970–86 (1993).

Grossarth-Maticek, Ronald, Jan Bastiaans, and Dusan T. Kanazir. "Psychosocial Factors as Strong Predictors of Mortality from Cancer, Ischaemic Heart Disease, and Stroke: The Yugoslav Prospective Study." 29 *Journal of Psychosomatic Research* 167–76 (1985).

Grossarth-Maticek, Ronald, Johannes Siegrist, and Hermann Vetter. "Interpersonal Repression as a Predictor of Cancer." 16 *Social Science and Medicine* 493–98 (1982).

Guthrie, George M., Anne Verstraete, Melissa M. Deines, et al. "Symptoms of Stress in Four Societies." 95 *Journal of Social Psychology* 165–72 (1975).

Hammett, Frederick S. "Studies of the Thyroid Apparatus: I." 56 *American Journal of Physiology* 196–204 (1921).

———. "Studies of the Thyroid Apparatus: V." 6 *Endocrinology* 221–29 (1922).

Hawkins, Anne Hunsaker. *Reconstructing Illness: Studies in Pathography.* West Lafayette, IN: Purdue University Press, 1993.

Helman, Cecil G. *Culture, Health and Illness: An Introduction for Health Professionals,* 2nd ed. London: Butterworth, 1990.

———. *Culture, Health and Illness: An Introduction for Health Professionals,* 3rd ed. London: Butterworth, 1994.

Holmes, T.H., and Masuda, M. "Life Change and Illness Susceptibility, Separation, and Depression." AAAS 161–86 (1973).

Idler, E. "Self-Assessed Health and Mortality: A Review of Studies." In *International Review of Health Psychology,* Vol. 1. S. Maes, et al. eds. New York: John Wiley, 1992.

Jamison, Kay Redfield. *An Unquiet Mind: A Memoir of Moods and Madness.* New York: Alfred A. Knopf, 1995.

Johnson, Jeffrey V., Walter Stewart, and Ellen M. Hall. "Long-Term Psychosocial Work Environment and Cardiovascular Mortality among Swedish Men." 86 *American Journal of Public Health* 324–31 (March 1996).

Justice, Blair. *Who Gets Sick: Thinking and Health.* Houston: Peak Press, 1987.

Kabat-Zinn, Jon. *Full Catastrophe Living: Using the Wisdom of Your Body and Mind to Face Stress, Pain, and Illness.* New York: Delacorte Press, 1990.

Kaplan, Sherrie, and Sheldon Greenfield. "Enlarging Patient Responsibility." *Forum: Risk Management Foundation of the Harvard Medical Institutions* 9–11 (1993).

Karasek, Robert A., R. Scott Russell, and Tores Theorell. "Physiology of Stress and Regeneration in Job-Related Cardiovascular Illness." 8 *Journal of Human Stress* 29–42 (March 1982).

Kiecolt-Glaser, J.K., and R. Glaser. "Psychosocial Moderators of Immune Function." 9 *Annals of Behavioral Medicine* 16–20 (1987).

Kissen, D.M. "Personality and Lung Cancer." 1 *Lancet* 216–17 (1964).

Kleinman, Arthur. *Patients and Healers in the Context of Culture: An Exploration of the Borderland Between Anthropology, Medicine and Psychiatry.* Berkeley: University of California Press, 1980.

Kleinman, Arthur, and Byron Good, eds. *Culture and Depression: Studies in the Anthropology and Cross-Cultural Psychiatry of Affect and Disorder.* Berkeley: University of California Press, 1985.

Kleinman, Arthur, and Joan Kleinman. "Somatization: The Interconnections in Chinese Society among Culture, Depressive Experiences, and the Meanings of Pain." In *Culture and Depression: Studies in the Anthropology and Cross-Cultural Psychiatry of Affect and Disorder.* A. Kleinman and B. Good, eds. Berkeley: University of California Press, 1985, pp. 429–90.

Kobasa, Suzanne C. "Stressful Life Events, Personality, and Health: An Inquiry into Hardiness." 37 *Journal of Personality and Social Psychology* 1–11 (Jan. 1979).

Krystal, Henry. "Alexithymia and Psychotherapy." 33 *American Journal of Psychotherapy* 17–31 (Jan. 1979).

Landis, Suzanne E., Victor J. Schoenbach, David J. Weber, et al. "Results of a

Randomized Trial of Partner Notification in Cases of HIV Infection in North Carolina." 326 *New England Journal of Medicine* 101–6 (Jan. 9, 1992).

Langer, Ellen. *The Psychology of Control*. Beverly Hills, CA: Sage, 1983.

Lau, Bernard W.K., Noel Y.T. Kung, and Joseph T.C. Chung. "How Depressive Illness Presents in Hong Kong." 227 *Practitioner* 112–14 (1983).

Lederer, Bob, with Kathy DeLeon. "The Newest AIDS Treatment Is Not a Drug." *POZ*, 62–65, 75 (Dec. 1995/Jan. 1996).

Leigh, Hoyle, and Morton F. Reiser. *The Patient: Biological, Psychological and Social Dimensions of Medical Practice*. New York: Plenum, 1980.

Lexchin, Joel. "Enforcement of Codes Governing Pharmaceutical Promotion: What Happens When Companies Breach Advertising Guidelines?" 156 *Canadian Medical Association Journal* 351–56 (Feb. 1, 1997).

Lipkin, Mark, and Gerri S. Lamb. "The Couvade Syndrome: An Epidemiological Study." 96 *Annals of Internal Medicine* 509–11 (1982).

Lynch, James J. *The Broken Heart: The Medical Consequences of Loneliness*. New York: Basic Books, 1977.

———. *The Language of the Heart: The Body's Response to Human Dialogue*. New York: Basic Books, 1985.

Maddi, Salvatore R., and Suzanne C. Kobasa. *The Hardy Executive: Health under Stress*. Homewood, IL: Dow Jones-Irwin, 1984.

Marx, J. "Anxiety Peptide Found in Brain." 227 *Science* 934 (1985).

Mayne, Tracy J., Eric Vittinghoff, Margaret A. Chesney, et al. "Depressive Affect and Survival among Gay and Bisexual Men Infected with HIV." 156 *Archives of Internal Medicine* 2233–38 (Oct. 28, 1996).

McClelland, David C. "Sources of Stress in the Drive for Power." In *Psychopathology of Human Adaptation*. G. Serban, ed. New York: Plenum, 1976, pp. 247–70.

McClintock, Martha K. "Menstrual Synchrony and Suppression." 229 *Nature* 244–45 (Jan. 22, 1971).

McCusker, Jane, Anne M. Stoddard, Kenneth H. Mayer, et al. "Effects of HIV Antibody Test Knowledge on Subsequent Sexual Behaviors in a Cohort of Homosexually Active Men." 78 *American Journal of Public Health* 462–67 (April 1988).

McGee, Rob, Sheila Williams, and Mark Elwood. "Depression and the Development of Cancer: A Metaanalysis." 38 *Social Science and Medicine* 187–92 (1994).

Meijer, Anne Marie, Rupino W. Griffioen, Jan C. van Nierop, et al. "Intractable or Uncontrollable Asthma: Psychosocial Factors." 32 *Journal of Asthma* 265–74 (1995).

Miller, Glenn A., and William Nuessle. "Characteristics of the Emotional Responsiveness of Sensitizers and Repressors to Social Stimuli." 46 *Journal of Consulting and Clinical Psychology* 339–40 (April 1978).

Montagu, Ashley. *The Direction of Human Development*, new and revised ed. New York: Hawthorn Books, 1970.

Moses, Leon, George E. Daniels, and John L. Nickerson. "Psychogenic Factors in Essential Hypertension: Methodology and Preliminary Report." 18 *Psychosomatic Medicine* 471–85 (1956).

Moyers, Bill. *Healing and the Mind*. New York: Doubleday, 1993.

Muller, James E., Paul L. Ludmer, Stefan N. Willich, et al. "Circadian Variation in the Frequency of Sudden Cardiac Death." 75 *Circulation* 131–38 (Jan. 1987).

Myers, David G. *The Pursuit of Happiness: Who Is Happy—and Why*. New York: William Morrow, 1992.

Narsavage, Georgia L. "Promoting Function in Clients with Chronic Lung Disease by Increasing Their Perception of Control." 12 *Holistic Nursing Practice* 17–26

(1997).

Nordstrom, Carolyn R. "Ayurveda: A Multilectic Interpretation." 28 *Social Science and Medicine* 963–70 (1989).

Okun, Morris A., William A. Stock, Marilyn J. Haring, et al. "Health and Subjective Well-Being: A MetaAnalysis." 19 *International Journal of Aging and Human Development* 111–32 (1994).

Ots, Thomas. "The Angry Liver, the Anxious Heart and the Melancholy Spleen: The Phenomenology of Perceptions in Chinese Culture." 14 *Culture, Medicine & Psychiatry* 21–58 (March 1990).

Parkes, C. Murray, B. Benjamin, and R.G. Fitzgerald. "Broken Heart: A Statistical Study of Increased Mortality among Widowers." 1 *British Medical Journal* 740–43 (March 22, 1969).

Pellegrine, Robert J. "Repression-Sensitizations and Perceived Severity of Presenting Problem of Four Hundred and Forty-Four Counseling Center Clients." 18 *Journal of Counseling Psychology* 332–36 (July 1971).

Pelletier, Kenneth. *Mind as Healer, Mind as Slayer: A Holistic Approach to Preventing Stress Disorders*. New York: Delta, 1977.

Pennebaker, James W., ed. *Emotion, Disclosure and Health*. Washington, DC: American Psychological Association, 1995(a).

Pennebaker, James W. "Emotional Disclosure and Health: An Overview." In *Emotion, Disclosure and Health*. Washington, DC: American Psychological Association, 1995(b), pp. 3–10.

Peterson, Christopher, Steven F. Maier, and Martin E.P. Seligman. *Learned Helplessness: A Theory for the Age of Personal Control*. New York: Oxford University Press, 1993.

Pfeiffer, W. "The Symptomatology of Depression Viewed Transculturally." 5 *Transcultural Psychiatric Research* 121–23 (1968).

Ports, Suki. "Needed (for Women and Children)." In *AIDS: CulturalAnalysis/Cultural Activism*. D. Crimp, ed. Cambridge: MIT Press, 1988, pp. 169–76.

Price, Reynolds. *A Whole New Life*. New York: Atheneum, 1994.

Rabkin, Judith G., Robert Remien, Lewis S. Katoff, et al. "Resilience in Adversity among Long-Term Survivors of AIDS." 44 *Hospital and Community Psychiatry* 162–67 (Feb. 1993).

Rabkin, Judith G., Robert Remien, and Christopher Wilson. *Good Doctors, Good Patients: Partners in HIV Treatment*. New York: NCM Publishers, 1994.

Rabkin, Judith G., Glenn Wagner, and Richard Rabkin. "Prevalence and Treatment of Depressive Disorders in HIV Illness." 2 *Medscape Mental Health* (1997) (see http://www.medscape.com/Medscape/MentalH...997/v02.n03/mh60.rabkin/mh60.rabkin.html).

Rabkin, Simon W., Francis A.L. Mathewson, and Robert B. Tate. "Chronobiology of Sudden Cardiac Death in Men." 244 *Journal of the American Medical Association* 1357–58 (Sept. 1980).

Reiser, Morton F., Milton Rosenbaum, and Eugene B. Ferris. "Psychologic Mechanisms and Malignant Hypertension." 13 *Psychosomatic Medicine* 147–59 (May/June 1951).

Rodin, Judith, and Peter Salovey. "Health Psychology." 40 *Annual Review of Psychology* 533–79 (1989).

Rogers, Carl R. *On Becoming a Person: A Therapist's View of Psychotherapy*. Boston: Houghton Mifflin, 1961.

Sachs, Robert. *Health for Life: Secrets of Tibetan Ayurveda*. Santa Fe, NM: Clear Light Publishers, 1995.

Sales, Stephen M., and James House. "Job Dissatisfaction as a Possible Risk Factor in Coronary Heart Disease." 23 *Journal of Chronic Disease* 861–73 (1971).

Schleifer, Steven J., Steven E. Keller, Maria Camerino, et al. "Suppression of Lymphocyte Stimulation Following Bereavement." 250 *Journal of the American Medical Association* 374–77 (1983).

Schwartz, Gary E. "Psychobiology of Repression and Health: A Systems Approach." In *Repression and Dissociation*. J.L. Singer, ed. Chicago: University of Chicago Press, 1990, pp. 405–34.

Seeman, Melvin, and Teresa E. Seeman. "Health Behavior and Personal Autonomy: A Longitudinal Study of the Sense of Control in Illness." 24 *Journal of Health and Social Behavior* 144–60 (June 1983).

Shankar, Darshan, and Ram Manohar. "Ayurveda Today—Ayurveda at the Crossroads." In *Oriental Medicine: An Illustrated Guide to the Asian Arts of Healing*. J. Van Alphen and A. Aris, eds. Boston: Shambhala, 1996, pp. 98–105.

Shekelle, Richard B., William J. Raynor, Adrian M. Ostfeld, et al. "Psychological Depression and 17-Year Risk of Death from Cancer." 43 *Psychosomatic Medicine* 117–25 (April 1981).

Shweder, Richard A. "Menstrual Pollution, Soul Loss, and the Comparative Study of Emotions." In *Culture and Depression: Studies in the Anthropology and Cross-Cultural Psychiatry of Affect and Disorder*. A. Kleinman and B. Good, eds. Berkeley: University of California Press, 1985, pp. 182–215.

Siegel, Bernie S. *Love, Medicine and Miracles: Lessons Learned about Self-Healing from a Surgeon's Experience with Exceptional Patients*. New York: Harper & Row, 1986.

————. *Peace, Love and Healing: Bodymind Communication and the Path to Self-Healing: An Exploration*. New York: Harper & Row, 1989.

Sifneos, Peter E. "The Prevalence of Alexithymic Characteristics in Psychosomatic Patients." 22 *Psychotherapy and Psychosomatics* 255–62 (1973).

Singer, Jerome L., and Julie B. Sincoff. "Summary Chapter: Beyond Repression and the Defenses." In *Repression and Dissociation: Implications for Personality Theory, Psychopathology and Health*. J.L. Singer, ed. Chicago: University of Chicago Press, 1990, pp. 471–96.

Singer, June. *Boundaries of the Soul: The Practice of Jung's Psychology*. New York: Anchor, 1972.

Smith, James Monroe. *AIDS and Society*. Upper Saddle River, NJ: Prentice-Hall, 1996.

————. "When Knowing the Law Is Not Enough: Confronting Denial and Considering Sociocultural Issues Affecting HIV Positive People." 17 *Hamline Journal of Public Law & Policy* 1–39 (Fall 1995).

Spiegel, David, Joan R. Bloom, Helena C. Kraemer, et al. "Effects of Psychosocial Treatment on Survival of Patients with Metastatic Breast Cancer." *Lancet* 888–91 (Oct. 15, 1989).

Spitz, René. "The Role of Ecological Factors in Emotional Development." 20 *Child Development* 145–55 (1949).

Spring, Richard, and Prabha Khanna. "Locus of Control, Repression Sensitization, and Interpersonal Causality." 50 *Psychological Reports* 175–97 (1982).

Storr, Anthony. *Solitude: A Return to the Self*. New York: Free Press, 1988.

Svoboda, Robert. "Theory and Practice of Ayurvedic Medicine." In *Oriental Medicine: An Illustrated Guide to the Asian Arts of Healing*. J. Van Alphen and A. Aris, eds. Boston: Shambhala, 1996, pp. 67–97.

Taylor, Shelley E. "Adjustment to Threatening Events: A Theory of Cognitive Adaptation." 38 *American Psychologist* 1161–73 (Nov. 1983).

Temoshok, Lydia. "Personality, Coping Style, Emotion and Cancer: Toward an Integrative Model." 6 *Cancer Surveys* 545–67 (1987).

Tseng, Wen-shing. "The Nature of Somatic Complaints among Psychiatric Patients." 16 *Comprehensive Psychiatry* 237–45 (1975).

Voelker, Rebecca. "Ames Agrees with Mom's Advice: Eat Your Fruits and Vegetables." 273 *Journal of the American Medical Association* 1077–78 (April 12, 1995).

———. "Nocebos Contribute to Host of Ills." *Journal of the American Medical Association* 345, 347 (Feb. 7, 1996).

Wakefield, Dan. *Expect a Miracle: The Miraculous Things That Happen to Ordinary People.* San Francisco: HarperSan Francisco, 1995.

Wang, Jen-Yi. "Psychosomatic Illness in the Chinese Cultural Context." In *The Anthropology of Medicine: From Culture to Method.* L. Romanucci-Ross, D.E. Moerman, and L.R. Tancredi, eds. South Hadley, MA: Bergin & Garvey, 1983, pp. 298–318.

Webster's New Collegiate Dictionary. Springfield, MA: G. & C. Merriam, 1981.

Webster's Third New International Dictionary. Springfield, MA: G. & C. Merriam, 1971.

Weeks, David Joseph, and Jamie James. *Eccentrics: A Study of Sanity and Strangeness.* New York: Villard, 1995.

Wegner, Daniel M., Joann W. Shortt, Anne W. Blake, et al. "The Suppression of Exciting Thoughts." 58 *Journal of Personality and Social Psychology* 409–18 (1990).

Weil, Andrew. *Spontaneous Healing: How to Discover and Enhance Your Body's Natural Ability to Maintain and Heal Itself.* New York: Alfred A. Knopf, 1995.

Weinberger, Daniel A. "The Construct Validity of the Repressive Coping Style." In *Repression and Dissociation: Implications for Personality Theory, Psychopathology and Health.* J.L. Singer, ed. Chicago: University of Chicago Press, 1990, pp. 337–86.

Weinberger, Daniel A., Gary E. Schwartz, and R.J. Davidson. "Low-Anxious, High-Anxious, and Repressive Coping Styles: Psychometric Patterns and Behavioral and Physiological Responses to Stress." 88 *Journal of Abnormal Psychology* 369–80 (1979).

Weiner, Herbert M. *Psychobiology of Essential Hypertension.* New York: Elsevier, 1979.

Wilkes, Michael S., Bruce H. Doblin, and Martin F. Shapiro. "Pharmaceutical Advertisements in Leading Medical Journals: Experts' Assessments." 116 *Annals of Internal Medicine* 912–19 (June 1, 1992).

Wolf, Stewart. "The Pharmacology of Placebos." 11 *Pharmacological Reviews* 689–704 (1959).

Yelin, Edward, Michael Nevitt, and Wallace Epstein. "Toward an Epidemiology of Work Disability." 58 *Milbank Memorial Fund Quarterly* 386–415 (1980).

5

The Role of the Spirit
in Health

INTRODUCTION

The profession of medicine appears to ignore the human spirit.

Eric J. Cassell,
"The Nature of Suffering and the Goals of Medicine," p. 643

This chapter attempts to define the "spirit" and explores how it is nourished and compromised. Religious and psychological aspects of our spirit world are also considered. Examining the religious dimensions of spirituality entails considering the many ways in which patients suffer and how this suffering can be lessened or alleviated and considering the power of prayer in our lives.

Psychological dimensions of our spirit world include our gifts of intuition and our ability to affirm others—to acknowledge their goodness to enable them to become the persons they are capable of becoming. We may also use our unconscious mind to contribute to our health. We allow ourselves to experience more emotional growth when we make the unconscious mind conscious—when we become aware of and then overcome the things we have repressed (Frankl, 1957, p. 4). There is also some evidence that one of the purposes of our unconscious mind is to lead us toward wholeness.

Illness need not damage or diminish our spirit; in fact, tragedy often enhances it. Some refer to this quality of spiritual strength as courage (Manske, 1990, p. 67). As Plutarch said, "The measure of a man is the way he bears up under misfortune" (Frankl, 1975, p. 126).

There is evidence that developing or embracing our spirit will enhance our health and give us the confidence to make choices about the direction of our lives. This increases our motivation to do the things consistent with who we are (see Langer, 1989, p. 85) and quite possibly promotes health.

DIFFERENT DEFINITIONS OF OUR SPIRIT

Several authors have pointed out that we are not defined by our physical bodies but by our spirits or souls (Weiss, 1995, p. 64). This chapter considers many different definitions of the spirit. It

- includes our higher power;
- is reflected by our values and virtues (Kushner, 1995, p. 21);
- is reflected by our capacity to create (Bolen, 1995, p. 4);
- is manifest in our awareness and ability to see beauty in the world (ibid., p. 8);
- includes the acceptance of what is (Siegel, 1986, p. 177); and
- is demonstrated by our involvement with life (Sanford, 1977, p. 19).

The Spirit as Including Our Higher Power and Awareness

Many have said that the spirit includes our higher power or is evidence of the divine in us. Some have also said that the divine speaks to us through our intuition (Buber, 1966; Vardey, 1995).

Carl Jung believed that the conscious will of individuals cannot be controlled when affected by conditions like addiction. In other words, human beings can be dominated by influences antagonistic to their deeper meaning and purposes (Kelsey, 1995, p. 51).

Knowledge alone will not enable persons to conquer their addictions. For example:

- Knowing that one does not need to have and should not have another drink does not stop the alcoholic from taking that drink.
- Being ashamed of one's behavior—of being addicted to sex—does not necessarily change one's habits of engaging in promiscuous and/or anonymous sex. Persons who habitually go to bars to pick up women or men solely for sexual intercourse may wish to change their behavior and vow to develop relationships through dating. They may believe that these latter relationships are more fulfilling and this fulfillment may be what they want out of life. Although they may go to a bar intending to look for a date, their best intentions can be set aside in the course of talking with someone in the bar, particularly as their addiction becomes further "enabled" by drinking alcohol.

Many believe that addictions can only be properly treated when addicts turn over their lives to a spiritual force. Since our awareness in enhanced when we learn to accept ourselves as we are (not what we'd like to be, think we should be, nor others would like us to be), it is quite possible that this awareness evokes our higher power.

The 12-step programs appear to some to be so effective because individuals share personal stories of their weaknesses (and the weaknesses they have overcome) (see Harrison, 1997, pp. 13–14). But to reveal our weaknesses, we must be honest with ourselves—and this honesty will come from our awareness.

The Spirit as Reflected by Our Virtues

Our virtues enable us to do good in the world and, consequently, are the manifestation of our spirit. For example, our courage (a virtue) is part of our spirit and is often manifest by the passion with which we address issues. And only with passion are we motivated to accomplish worthy ends.

The Spirit as Reflected by Our Capacity to Create

The soul is the sense of something higher than ourselves, something that stirs in us thoughts, hopes, and aspirations which go out to the world of goodness, truth, and beauty.

Albert Schweitzer,
Reverence for Life, p. 78

Being in touch with our spirit allows us to forge our own journey and not to imitate another's path. By forging our journey, we become aware that we can make choices and become responsible for our decisions.

To forge our unique journey, however, we must be creative. Only we can determine what our unique mark on the world will be. But to be creative, we must not feel constrained by social norms—for in being what we think others may expect of us, we may fail to be true to ourselves.

The Spirit as Manifest in Our Awareness of Beauty

Spirituality may be the ability to see beauty in the world (Bolen, 1995). Our ability to perceive beauty is spiritual because we must use our awareness to have new insights or even to see the physical world in a different way. This awareness may also involve realization that we are all walking different paths to the same end, that we have more in common because we are all human. When we develop this awareness, we may have greater compassion for each other.

The Spirit as the Acceptance of What Is

Bernie Siegel has defined spirituality as the "acceptance of what is" (Siegel, 1986, p. 177); this concept is similar to Scott Peck's notion that we must remain dedicated to reality at all costs (Peck, 1983, p. 162).

Siegel is quite likely saying that if we learn to live with our illness and if we learn to love ourselves, then we will respond to our illness in a positive way. If our illnesses do not get in the way of living, we have responded to them in a positive manner. This interpretation is consistent with Siegel's notion that "we bring meaning [into our lives] by how we love the world" (Siegel, 1993, p. 5).

The Spirit as Demonstrated by Our Involvement with Life

Our spirit reflects the measure of our involvement with life (Sanford, 1977, p. 19). That involvement is certainly related to our ability to commit ourself to something—a requirement that Viktor Frankl believed to be necessary to establish our identity (Frankl, 1967, p. 180).

HOW THE SPIRIT IS NOURISHED

The spirit is nourished through many means, including

- communicating with others, which enhances our friendships and ability to have meaningful and intimate relationships (Cassell, 1982, p. 643; Moore, 1995, p. 27);
- forgiving others (Borysenko, 1995, p. 45; Gray, 1995, p. 56): It has been said, "To hold a grudge is like carrying the devil on your shoulders" (Banks, 1995, p. 77);
- serving others (Borysenko, 1995, p. 45);
- committing ourselves to action that has truth and integrity (Fulghum, 1995, p. 10): Such action includes our commitment to overcome our problems, such as our addictions (Kushner, 1995, p. 23);
- practicing, among others, the values of love, courage, patience, compassion, generosity, and wisdom (Gray, 1995, p. 56);
- learning to find holiness in unholy situations, such as in the activities of our daily lives (Kushner, 1995, p. 18);
- revering our own lives (Branden, 1995, p. 103);
- reaching for the best within ourselves (ibid.); and
- accepting our lot: Many people who experience sudden breakthroughs in health "do not expend energy on being bitter, resentful, and angry for the hand they have been dealt" (Dossey, 1991, p. 197); they refuse to be "victims" and they do things that will support their being and spirit.

Our spirituality, or the beauty within us, therefore, may be "released" through nonverbal forms, such as painting, dance, or music. Music therapy, for example, is increasingly recognized for its capacity to elicit profound healing responses (Dossey, 1991; see also Campbell, 1992). In one case, an 11-year-old diagnosed with catatonic schizophrenia had not uttered a word in seven years (Dossey, 1991, p. 145). But when his therapist played Bach's "Jesu, Joy of Man's Desiring," the boy began to weep and sobbed through his tears, "That is the most powerful music I have ever heard; now I can speak" (ibid.)!

HOW THE SPIRIT IS COMPROMISED

Introduction

I protest on behalf of who I am and so that my spirit might live on.
                                                      Dietrich Bonhoeffer,
                                                      quoted in Sinetar,
                                                      Living Happily Ever After, p. 163

Dietrich Bonhoeffer, German pastor and Christian martyr executed by the Nazis, was willing to die for what he believed was just—it was more important for him to preserve his spirit and his ideals than his body. As a result, he left us a legacy of courage and conviction. He suggests that we compromise our spirit by being unwilling to die for a cause. The ultimate test of the strength of our spirit is our ability to shed our fear of death and to act and speak consistently with who we are. Although it is unrealistic to expect that most people will become martyrs in order to preserve their integrity and spirit, the lesson learned from Bonhoeffer is profound. There were not many who were willing to challenge the Nazis because they were immobilized by fear of death or persecution.

Some may see it as odd to quote Bonhoeffer in a book about health. But Bonhoeffer has shown us how important it is to develop peace of mind by taking steps consistent with our beliefs. Our capacity to develop peace of mind may depend upon our ability to develop courage and to assert who and what we are. This will require us to reject concerns about what others think of us. When we choose to be honest and state our beliefs, hopes, and dreams, we enhance our spirit and soul. In the world of psychology and psychiatry this is called becoming *authentic* or *self-actualized* (a term of Abraham H. Maslow) (Maslow, 1968). Unfortunately, as illustrated in the highlight box, "Living A Lie—Adolescent Women," many people are socialized to "live a lie" and to relinquish their authentic selves.

The psychiatrist Erich Fromm suggests that we compromise our spirit when we become "indifferent to life," as when we lose our capacity to be moved by the distress of another (Fromm, 1964, p. 150). We become indifferent to life because of the accumulated wrong choices we have made (ibid.). Fromm says that many people

are not aware when life asks them a question, and when they still have alternative answers. Then with each step along the wrong road it becomes increasingly difficult for them to admit that they are on the wrong road, often only because they have to admit that they must go back to the first wrong turn, and must accept the fact that they have wasted time and energy. (ibid., p. 138)

How Evil Compromises the Spirit

The human spirit is suppressed through human evil (see Peck, 1983, p. 42). The psychiatrists Erich Fromm and M. Scott Peck have described the characteristics of the evil person, who may

* scapegoat or put down others (ibid., p. 129);
* not tolerate criticism and other forms of narcissistic injury (ibid). Because of their narcissism, the evil do not consider a situation from another's viewpoint because they lack empathy (ibid., p. 136);
* be excessively concerned with their public image;

LIVING A LIE—ADOLESCENT WOMEN

When adolescent women choose to be socially accepted, they "split into two selves, one that is authentic and one that is culturally scripted" (Pipher, 1994, p. 38). This "cultural script" causes young women to feel that their intelligence is a liability and they feel pressured to be feminine instead of whole, and popular instead of honest (ibid., p. 255). In giving up their honesty, girls become uncomfortable identifying and stating their needs (especially with boys and adults) (ibid., p. 257).

The problems that adolescent women face have recently been brought to the public's attention with the publication of two major works: the American Association of University Women's Study, *How Schools Shortchange Girls* [*The AAUW Report*] (1992) and Mary Pipher's best-seller, *Reviving Ophelia* (1994).

Women and Self-Esteem

Most research indicates that during the elementary school years, there are no differences in self-esteem in males and females (Simmons & Rosenberg, 1975). However, during adolescence females begin to score lower than males on measures of self-esteem (Cairns, McWhirter, Duffy, et al., 1990). But girls' self-esteem benefits if there is only one transition at the end of the eighth grade rather than two changes: first, from elementary school to middle school or junior high school, then from there to high school (*The AAUW Report*, 1992, p. 13). Some believe that the decline in self-esteem for young women may be due to

- their awareness of the lower status society places on "relationship tending" and the higher status it places on autonomy and independence (Chubb, Fertman, & Ross, 1997).
- the different amounts and types of reinforcement young women receive from teachers (ibid.): Studies show that, in the classroom, boys are called on more frequently than girls (*The AAUW Report*, p. 68); receive more precise teacher comments (ibid., p. 69); are asked more abstract, complex, and open-ended questions; are 12 times more likely to speak up in class; and have more classroom activities that appeal to them (Pipher, 1994, p. 62).
- negative messages that young girls receive through the school curriculum (*The AAUW Report*, 1992, p. 67): A 1971 study of

13 popular United States history texts showed that material on women totaled no more than 1 percent of any text (ibid., *citing* Trecker, 1971). The author of this study concluded that when women's lives were covered, they were "trivialized" or "distorted" (ibid.).

The self-esteem of young women is also affected by the beliefs that boys verbalize. As early as the eighth grade, boys believe that they are better leaders than girls, that families should encourage sons rather than daughters to attend college, and that girls should be more concerned with "becoming good wives and mothers" than pursuing a profession or business career (Boxley, Lawrance, & Gruchow, 1995).

Girls' self-esteem is also undermined by the verbal and physical harassment they receive from boys at school—50 percent of girls experience unwanted sexual touching at their schools and 25 percent of girls report being cornered and molested at school (*The AAUW Report*, 1992, pp. 69–70).

The "Liability" of Intelligence

Studies have shown that gifted girls actually lose IQ points as they become "feminized" (ibid., p. 63; Kerr, 1985, p. 103). There are many reasons that intelligence is seen as a "liability." Consider some of the following:

- Girls may begin to see their own giftedness as "undesirable" (Kerr, 1985, p. 103)—they hold back when they "have something to contribute" (ibid., p. 105).
- Girls' parents may worry about their attractiveness to boys (and, of course, the impact of their giftedness on their ability to enter "relationships") (ibid.).
- Smart girls are often the most rejected by their peers (ibid., p. 266; see also p. 19).

When boys fail, their failures are attributed to external factors; however, girls' failure is attributed to lack of ability (ibid., p. 63). Therefore, with each successive "failure," girls' confidence is eroded (ibid.). This loss of confidence is suggested by the fact that girls are more likely than boys to admit that they "are not smart enough for their dream careers" (ibid.). Furthermore, competent females have higher expectations of failure and lower self-confidence when encountering new academic situations than do males with similar abilities (Lenney, 1977).

- be intellectually devious and dishonest (ibid.), not likely disclose their true nature either to others or to themselves (ibid., p. 104);
- be surprisingly obedient to authority (ibid., p. 180);
- be greedy (ibid., p. 72);
- make others dependent upon them—evil persons seek to control others (Fromm, 1964, p. 41);
- discourage others from thinking for themselves—and we think for ourselves when we make choices. Thinking for ourselves thus ensures our capacity to be free (see ibid., p. 136); and
- suppress another's originality (ibid.): As Fromm has said, "The man who cannot create wants to destroy" (ibid., p. 31).

How Our Desires Compromise the Spirit

Gandhi once said that modern civilization involves "an indefinite multiplicity of human wants" (Attenborough, 1982, p. 17). He believed that it was in humankind's best interest to reduce the number of its wants. He knew that individuals cannot fully satisfy their desires—that the more goods they have, the more goods they want to consume. Because of this never-ending cycle, we can become solely focused on the consumption of goods and the satisfaction of our wants, not reserving the time needed for proper spiritual, emotional, and psychological development.

Since illness often affects people's ability to work, it is almost inevitably associated with financial repercussions. In our society, therefore, sick people generally do not consume as many goods as the more healthy do. As a result, sick people may use their free time for other positive pursuits, such as personal reflection and spiritual, psychological, and emotional development.

DISEASES OF THE SPIRIT

Psychologists have referred to both suicide and alcoholism as spiritual problems (Sanford, 1977, p. 25). The use of alcohol, for example, is associated with turbulent emotions such as anxiety, depression, or overwhelming guilt (Zeller, 1967, p. 267). Consider the following case report, which details the psychological/spiritual struggle of one individual who committed suicide.

SUICIDE: A CASE EXAMPLE

A Nazi fighter pilot was referred to a Jungian analyst for treatment because he developed hysterical color blindness—he could see everything in black and white even though there was nothing organically wrong with his vision (see Sanford, 1977, p. 13). He saw the situation in Germany during the rise of Hitler and during the war as black and white too: "Everything that was useful to

Germany, Hitler and the victory, was good; everything else was bad" (ibid.). The patient adored his brother, who was a member of the SS, and hated his sister, who he considered to be a traitor because she had joined the resistance (ibid).

The pilot reported his dreams were "reversed from the way [they] should have been" (ibid., p. 14). He dreamed that his brother, "dressed in an SS uniform, had a uniform that was white and a black face" and that his sister was "dressed in black prison garb, but her face was shining white" (ibid.).

Although the pilot thought that his dreams "changed everything around," he apparently made an important comment about the uniforms: he said that "the outside appearance does not matter; it's the face that's important" (ibid.). The analyst said that this differentiation was significant, for the pilot recognized the distinction between the outside and the inside, "between the persona expressing the outside reality, and the face, the expression of inside reality" (ibid.).

Some time after these dreams, the pilot was with his brother, who in a drunken state described what went on in the concentration camps (ibid.). That night the pilot dreamed, "a long column of concentration camp inmates with radiant white faces marched past Hitler. Hitler's face was black and he raised his hand, the color of which was the deep red color of blood" (ibid.).

The pilot expressed a desire to visit a concentration camp to find out for himself what went on there. One last note sent from the pilot to the analyst stated: "I believed too long that black was white. Now the many colors of the world won't help me anymore." Shortly after this note was sent, the pilot committed suicide.

Sanford concluded that the analyst "bravely aided the creative forces of the patient's own unconscious," and noted that consciousness inevitably broke through (ibid., pp. 14–15). But the consequences of the pilot's "newfound consciousness were intolerable" (ibid., p. 15). In other words, "[t]he annihilation of the old ego with its false beliefs, and the seeming impossibility of any longer existing in his Nazi Germany, were too much for him and he committed suicide" (ibid.). Sanford concludes that the young pilot committed suicide "because of health, but health was something the young man could not endure" (ibid.).

RELIGION, SPIRITUALITY, AND HEALTH

> It is clear that spiritual healing does not have the same focus as medicine and psychology. For its perspective, which has not evolved from the scientific method, does not refer only to what one is, but to what one can be.
>
> John T. Chirban,
> "Healing and Spirituality," in *Health and Faith*, pp. 10–11

Religions frequently provide a context in which to practice our spirituality, although one need not be religious or associated with a formal religion in order to be spiritual. Spiritual people probably all come to see a "force" in the universe greater than they: to Native Americans the earth and all things in it (from rocks to people) deserve respect partly because "every object had a spirit" (Williams, 1986, p. 21).

Spiritual practices have been tapped for their capacity to heal. Native Americans used medicine men or shamans to heal people of physical and psychological wounds (Lyon, 1996).[1] And in Tibet monks are also doctors (Tsenam, 1996): in that country, there has never been the rigorous separation of spirituality and medicine that has occurred in the West. When reading about traditional Tibetan medicine, it is not unusual to find as much about compassion as about Tibetan scientific precepts (ibid.). Khenpo Trosu Tsenam, head of the Traditional Tibetan Medical Hospital in Lhasa, says that compassion includes "a quality of openness and sensitivity on the part of the healing physician concerning what is objectively happening in the patient" (ibid., p. 147).

Monk-physicians also recognize the mind/body connection. In fact, their view of compassion mandates awareness of what is happening in both the mind and body of the patient (ibid.). In their medical scheme, desire, anger, and ignorance are classified as the three poisons (ibid., p. 149).

Spirituality is also so powerful because it may enable us to find meaning in life. Einstein believed that through religion we could answer the question, "What is the meaning of life?" (Frankl, 1975, p. 13).

But to find meaning in life, we must experience life—and engage in the journey of looking, feeling, and learning. Gandhi, who referred to the "purity of the struggle," called upon our need to focus on the means by which we pursue our journey, not necessarily the ends we attain. Gandhi himself said, "Joy lies in the fight, in the attempt, in the suffering involved, not in the victory itself" (Attenborough, 1982, p. 13).

Any discussion of spirituality must also include discussion of where our spirituality should lead us. Many great leaders and spiritual persons have suggested that spirituality must involve us in a human rights movement in which we seek justice for those without rights. For Gandhi, this involved entering the realm of politics.

The Problem of Suffering

Commentators about spirituality often refer to the realm of suffering. Consequently, spirituality may enable those who suffer to learn how to deal with their suffering—how to cope more effectively, how to grow emotionally despite their suffering, or how to maintain their dignity in spite of all the difficulties they confront (Harrison, 1997). Frequently, suffering is associated with a loss of self-respect (Bulger, 1992, p. 54).

The Spectrum of Suffering. But suffering means different things to different people. As the following indicates, suffering frequently includes "injuries" such as powerlessness, helplessness, hopelessness, torture, the loss of a life's work, betrayal, memory failure, and fear (Cassell, 1982). For example, consider the many ways in which people may suffer:

- Some may suffer when they cannot have what they want (and those wants we'll assume are not necessities).
- Some may suffer because of limitations imposed by illness: Consequently, for an active person, immobility is a form of suffering (Braillier, 1992, p. 205).
- Some suffer when illness prevents them from realizing their goals.
- Others suffer when they cannot fully adjust to various psychological and physical losses.
- The elderly in nursing homes often suffer because they are deprived of choices in their lives—even in ordinary activities like when to eat, wake up, and go to the bathroom—and this lack of choice causes them to lose touch with the person they once were (Starck, 1992, p. 132).
- People suffer not only from disease, but from the treatments used to treat disease (Hunter, 1991): For example, chemotherapy frequently causes exhaustion, which, unrelieved by rest or sleep, can be considered a form of suffering (Braillier, 1992, p. 205).
- shame or humiliation may cause suffering, as when patients perceive their diseases to be defects, inadequacies, or shortcomings (Lazare, 1992, p. 227).

Some physicians have expressed a need for doctors to understand suffering (ibid). They have recognized that "the relief of suffering . . . is considered one of the primary ends of medicine by patients and lay persons, but not by the medical profession" (Cassell, 1982, p. 640).

Because the nature of suffering is broad, doctors may feel at a loss as to how they can address it. One physician has noted that "the bereaved are not all sad in the same way. . . . Some are sad for reasons that can be addressed" (Hunter, 1991, p. 159). Even if the reason for the patient's suffering cannot be addressed, "[m]any are stronger and healthier for having their sadness acknowledged" (ibid.).

Religious Explanations as to the Cause of Suffering. As discussed in chapter 3, religions have made "moral" pronouncements about the sick, believing that disease has been contracted through immorality. Religions often feel obligated to explain why some people get sick and others do not. Religions refuse to accept the uncertainty in life and the randomness and chaos that exist in the universe. Members of various religions believe that people suffer because

- they are being punished for their sins (Kushner, 1981, pp. 6–30): This paradigm mandates a perception that there is fairness in the universe and that one will be rewarded for one's good deeds or punished for one's evil deeds.
- they are being given suffering and sickness in order to be spiritually strengthened (ibid., pp. 28–30): Sickness exists to try human patience and, therefore, "enables the sufferer to grow in faith and become more saintly" (Kelsey, 1995, p. 16).
- they can "handle" it (ibid., p. 36–38): Moslems believe that "Allah knows what individuals can bear and metes out their suffering accordingly" (Heitman, 1992, pp. 90–91).
- suffering, in the view of Christianity, is related to being "sinfully human" (ibid., p. 89): The reason for suffering, which is part of God's "infinite mystery," will only be revealed at the Last Judgment (ibid., p. 90).

Religious Beliefs and Survival

Many studies are beginning to suggest that religious persons are healthier and that religious persons with certain diseases are less likely to die than nonreligious persons with the same disease (Christy, 1998; Jaret, 1998; Kark, Shemi, Friedlander, et al., 1996; Wallis, 1996). Conclusions from several studies follow.

- Heart patients who said they drew "comfort from their religious beliefs" were three times more likely to survive bypass surgery than those of "little faith" (Jaret, 1998). This 1995 study was based on data from 232 heart surgery patients and is one of the few to separate the effect of social support from religious conviction (Wallis, 1996). In fact, the study's authors found that study participants who had *both* strong religious convictions and social support were 14 times more likely to recover than those with little faith and few friends (Jaret, 1998).
- Death rates of men and women who attended "religious services regularly" were only 65 percent of those of people who rarely entered a church or synagogue (ibid.). In this study, 5,000 persons were tracked for 28 years.
- Statistics over 16 years, comparing 11 religious and 11 matched secular kibbutzim in Israel, showed a significantly lower mortality rate in the religious kibbutzim for all major causes of death (Kark, Shemi, Friedlander, et al., 1996).
- Those to whom religion was "very important" had lower diastolic blood pressure readings (by about 5 mm Hg) than those who did not (Wallis, 1996). This 1989 study of 400 patients was adjusted to account for smoking and other risk factors (ibid.). These observations have been confirmed by other studies (Koenig, George, Hays, et al., 1998 [those who attended religious services and prayed or studied the Bible frequently were 40 percent less likely to have a diastolic blood pressure of 90 mm Hg than those who attended religious services and studied the Bible infrequently]).
- Devout Mormons have had lower rates of cancer than less devout Mormons (Christy, 1998).
- Depression and anxiety are lower among the religiously committed (Wallis, 1996).

Some researchers have attempted to find a physiological basis for the differences in health of believers and nonbelievers (or churchgoers versus nonchurchgoers). One researcher has reported that the elderly who regularly attend religious services have lower blood levels of the chemical interleukin-6 (Koenig, Cohen, George, et al., 1997).

Some studies suggest that religious beliefs have an association with survival rate (Oxman, Freeman, & Manheimer, 1995). In one study, heart disease patients who had open heart surgery and had received "solace and comfort" from their religious beliefs were three times more likely to survive than patients who did not (ibid.).

Those with religious beliefs are often churchgoers. A review of 27 studies showed that in 22 of them there was a positive and statistically significant relationship between the frequency of religious service attendance and health (Levin & Vanderpool, 1989).

Prayer, Prayerfulness, and Health

Prayer is about "being mindful of the moment and perceiving the magic in the mundane" (Dossey, 1996, p. 98). But people pray through "the witness of their lives, through the work they do, the friendships they have, [and] the love they offer people and receive from people" (ibid, p. 127). The latter definition of prayer suggests that one does not have to believe in God in order to pray. Larry Dossey has noted that even agnostics are often spiritual (ibid., p. 42) and that Buddhists, who do not believe in a God, pray to the Universe (ibid., p. 82).

Some have defined prayerfulness as

- having an attitude or state of mind in which we feel a sacred connection with the Absolute (ibid.).
- accepting without being passive and being grateful without giving up (Dossey, 1993, p. 24).

These definitions suggest that prayer inspires hope. One author, who described a physician who prayed with his sick mother for over an hour, reported that "the doctor's spirituality gave all of them the perspective and hope to confront what was seemingly insurmountable—not to mention what it did for them physically" (Chirban, 1991, p. 10).

Prayer may promote healing by allowing patients to develop peace of mind and to experience hope, perhaps because they have felt renewed.

It is not unusual for doctors to pray for patients; some studies have indicated that 43 percent of American physicians do so (Dossey, 1996, p. 71; see Martin & Carlson, 1988). Nearly 50 percent of hospitalized patients in one study wanted their doctors not only to pray for them but to pray with them (ibid., p. 69).

PSYCHOLOGY AND THE SPIRIT

The heart has its reasons which reason cannot know.

Blaise Pascal,
Pensées

What is to give light must endure burning.

Wildgans
quoted in Frankl,
The Doctor and the Soul, p. 77

The Dynamics of Intuition

I have found that when I have trusted some inner non-intellectual sensing, I have discovered wisdom in the move.

Carl Rogers,
On Becoming a Person, p. 22

Intuition has been defined as

- "an attunement to information not perceived by most conscious minds" (Langer, 1989, p. 119).
- "a quick perception of a truth without conscious attention or reasoning" (Arnold, 1978, p. 19).
- part of us that "at a deep level knows the right way" (Siegel, 1993, p. xv).
- the means by which the divine speaks to us (Vardey, 1995, p. 20).

Two of these definitions suggest that intuition involves knowing the truth or right way (see also ibid., p. xv).

The Dynamics of the Unconscious Mind

Jung defined the unconscious as consisting of

everything of which I know, but of which I am not at the moment thinking; everything of which I was once conscious but have now forgotten; everything perceived by my senses, but not noted by my conscious mind; everything which involuntarily and without paying attention to it, I feel, think, remember, want, and do; all the future things that are taking shape in me and will sometime come to consciousness: all this is the content of the unconscious. (Jung, 1969, p. 185)

The nature of the unconscious mind is revealed to us in dreams, where "the precise language of science is replaced with the language of imagination" (Muff, 1996). The unconscious mind may function to produce wholeness (ibid.). Consequently, an individual's dreams are believed to

- challenge the dreamer to consider the urgency of unfinished business (dreams of this nature contain images of time passing) (ibid.).
- confront the dreamer to recognize "whatever forces oppose the waking ego" including resolving any conflict surrounding one's illness (Levitan, 1980).
- allow the psyche to "digest" the more disagreeable parts of ourselves.
- make us consider questions about the meaning of existence and to "see the bigger picture": Even for people confused in the wake of dementia, "their dreams showed that their psyche was aware of the larger issues" (ibid.).
- reveal "clues" that are relevant to the preservation of our health (see Kushi & Esko, 1996).

Some people have even reported being first aware of having an illness as a result of "clues" that occurred in dreams (Donnelly & McPeak, 1996). Consider this: a Portuguese citizen working in the United States was thinking about moving back to Portugal when he dreamed that he could not return because he was HIV-positive. Despite the fact that this gay man felt perfectly fine and had no symptoms, he obtained an HIV test, which detected that he was HIV-positive.

Using the Unconscious Mind to Assist Patients to Heal

Some doctors have used techniques—beginning with careful listening—to tap into the patient's unconscious mind in an effort to understand what illness means to the patient (Matthews, Suchman, & Branch, 1993). Unconscious process "will persistently urge the patient toward healing and growth and attempt to bring underlying problems to light, within the bounds of what the patient can accept consciously" (ibid., p. 974). In order to be able to "tap" the patient's unconscious, doctors must be aware that a patient's behavior (and words) is seldom random and "that there is information to be gained from noticing how things are said, what is said, and what remains unsaid" (ibid.). In the following case, the patient's treating physician was particularly sensitive to the way something was said—particularly to the metaphors the patient used.

The patient was a 56 year old man who was seen for follow-up for hypertension and depression. The patient was angry about his treatment from his employer and his hostile comments about the company he worked for "were peppered with references to being 'shot in the back,' 'stabbed in the back,' 'raped from behind.'" When the patient described himself as a veteran, his doctor encouraged him to describe his war experiences. The patient said, "I don't know whether I should tell you about this," then paused. His doctor asked him if he killed anyone. "His belligerent tone turned remorseful, and he spoke of deliberately shooting a teenage civilian in the back for no particular reason, other than that he had just downed a few drinks and had been dared to do it by one of his comrades." (ibid., pp. 974–75)

The Dynamics of Affirmation

> Sometimes it is necessary to reteach a thing its loveliness.
>
> Galway Kinnel
> quoted in *Courage to Change*, p. 67

When people's goodness is affirmed, they can blossom into the very person they have always been capable of becoming. To affirm another enhances the other's inmost spirit. As Ralph Waldo Emerson said, "Treat people greatly and they will show themselves great" (Emerson, 1983, p. 365).

Although people may know deep within that they are inherently good, sometimes they need to be reminded of their capacity to be good. Many people go though life with little affirmation (see Moyers, 1993, p. 155) of their spirit and with little reminder of what Galway Kinnel refers to as their "loveliness." To give this "loveliness" to another is to gift that person incalculably.

The Dynamics of Awareness

When we are more aware or mindful, we are more in touch, sometimes even filled, with our spirits. The mindfulness developed through meditation is believed to cultivate people's ability to trust (Kabat-Zinn, 1994, p. 58), be generous (ibid., p. 61), be disciplined (ibid., p. 181), be more aware of the choices available to them (ibid., p. 223), and appreciate peacefulness (ibid., p. 8).

CHAPTER SUMMARY

When defining the spirit, the religious term *soul* is often encountered. The spirit represents many things to many people. From a religious perspective, it includes our "higher power." It may include our virtues, capacity to create, awareness of beauty, acceptance of what is, and involvement with life.

The spirit may be nourished or compromised in many ways. We nourish our spirit through forgiving and serving others, committing ourselves to act with truth and integrity, reaching for the best within ourselves, and finding holiness in common daily activities. Evil, our desires, and certain diseases (alcoholism and suicide) compromise our spirits.

Religion and spirituality are closely connected—although persons may be spiritual but not religious. Often it is through a spiritual quest that we find meaning in life. But we must be aware that the journey that this quest may comprise is considered as important as is the destination. Gandhi reminded us to be aware of the "purity" of our struggle and to find joy in our journey.

The problem of suffering is intimately related to the topics of religion and spirituality. It is important to remember, however, that people suffer in different ways. Some suffer from the limitations imposed by illness—because these limitations may thwart their dreams and goals—and others suffer from the treatment used to cure disease. Persons in nursing homes suffer because they are deprived of choices in their lives and, as a result, lose touch with the persons they once were.

Suffering is considered the "most fundamental problem of religion," and, as a result, religions have attempted to find meaning in suffering. Some religions argue that those who suffer are being punished for their sins or behavior in this or a past life, are being tested spiritually, or are allowed to suffer because they can handle it. For Christians, suffering is believed to be related to being "sinfully human"; the mystery that explains our suffering will only be revealed at the Last Judgment.

Our unconscious mind, revealed in dreams, is believed to assist us in our journey toward healing and wholeness. Even the dreams of persons who are demented seem to show that their psyche remains aware of the "larger issues." Furthermore, our dreams may reveal "clues" related to preserving our health. Many report that our dreams may lead us to become aware, for the first time, of physical illness.

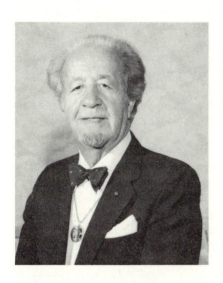

AN INTERVIEW WITH JOSEPH GELBERMAN

I am 86 years old. I've been trained as a rabbi and psychotherapist and I currently practice both professions. In connection with my rabbinical training, in 1971 I co-founded the New Seminary, an institute for the training of Interfaith Ministers who teach, counsel and work in the community. For example, such ministers learn how to: pray with people; visit the sick; conduct healing ceremonies, funerals, memorial services and weddings; and lead guided meditations. I am also currently the director of the Mid-way Counseling Center of New York City.

My entire family was annihilated in the Holocaust and I came to the United States in 1939. There must be an explanation for events as horrible as the Holocaust. I believe we must bury the past and not be consumed or victimized by it. Every day I remind myself that this is the day the Lord has made and that we must rejoice in it. We must not only savor each day, but each moment.

I would define spirituality as our awareness of our sacred responsibility to correct the evils in the universe and to realize our obligation to bring about peace and joy. God needs us here on earth. He does not need us in heaven because he has angels there! As he reminded Adam and Eve, he purposefully left the universe unfinished so that humans could leave their mark on it. Certainly that mark might be for good or evil.

In order to leave our personal mark on the universe, we must first change ourselves. We must not expect others to change themselves. We must not become emotionally overwrought by the evil or bad things others do—this depletes us and affects our capacity to do our work.

Religious persons practice the commandments and bring love and joy to the people they interact with. Faith requires that we act and, for example, do good works.

Most of the clients that I see in psychotherapy are searching for happiness and meaning in their lives. Since so many persons are dissatisfied with their jobs, I would advise them to "sanctify their work" and consider the opportunities that their work provides them (e.g., supporting their spouse and children). As Martin Buber said, the difference between the holy and unholy is that the unholy is waiting to be sanctified.

I believe that doctors should be spiritual. This would enable them to connect soul-to-soul with patients. At the New Seminary, we have a course for physicians called the "Physician of the Soul Program." In keeping with the New Seminary's philosophy of "Never Instead, Always in Addition," spiritual approaches to healing are not recommended to replace or substitute for conventional healing methods, such as medicine and psychotherapy. The course is intended to introduce methodologies that can serve as an adjunct and supplement for conventional practices.

I believe that effective doctors also need to be wise. To be wise is to know something about everything and to utilize it.

During our lives we each will experience light and darkness. We are not socialized to accept suffering and pain. Therefore, our challenge will be to learn how to accept the darkness that will visit us.

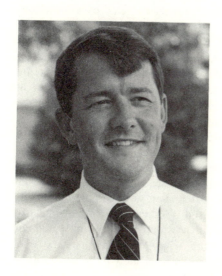

AN INTERVIEW WITH NIGEL MUMFORD

For the past three years, I have been the director of the Oratory of the Little Way, a Christian healing retreat center run under the auspices of the Episcopal Diocese of Connecticut. The Oratory is 1 of only 3 such residential healing centers in the United States, as compared to 33 such centers in England. It is a place where the walking wounded and spiritually dying can come for rest and renewal.

In my opinion, the biblical root of the healing ministry is to be found in James 5:14–16: "Is anyone among you sick? Let him call for the elders of the church. Let them pray with him, anointing him with oil, in the name of the Lord and the prayer of faith will save the sick and the Lord will raise him." This incorporates not only the laying on of hands and the forgiveness of sins, but also the commitment of the individual to seek not prayer but the wonder of answered prayer. I do not believe that one has to believe in God in order to be healed, but one does have to be willing to ask for healing. A mustard seed of faith is all that is necessary, and sometimes that mustard seed of faith can come from someone other than the person in need of healing. It may be that all the faith one needs is to pick up the car keys to drive to the healing center. To be healed emotionally, one must be able to forgive others. My sister, for example, was dramatically healed from a neurological condition that was misdiagnosed by her doctors, but her emotional condition could only heal after she forgave them.

It is important to understand that the power of prayer and the practice of medicine go hand in hand in terms of healing. I like people to consider the metaphor of the railroad tracks, the one being spiritual and the other medical. They are parallel and complementary tracks that are connected by railroad ties representing the days of our lives. When we look into the distance the tracks appear to come together. Yet when one of the rails is missing or damaged, the train cannot run. The harmony between our body and spirit is a question of balance and complementary parallels, and the care of both should be addressed. I believe that many times, people with cancer have experienced some sort of emotional trauma prior to the onset of their cancer. This belief echoes the Simontons' research [see their book referenced here] which shows that as many as 85 percent of persons with cancer suffered a trauma prior to the onset of the disease.

The foundation of my own healing ministry is simply to listen, love, and pray. When I meet with people, I listen to what they are saying, what they are not saying, and what God is saying. I make my prayer as specific as possible, visualizing the physical problem being repaired. Furthermore, I often find that the unspoken problems are at the core of that which is being presented for healing. I believe that prayer is communication with God on a very deep level and that the effects of prayer can be likened to those of the wind—although the wind cannot be seen, we realize its power and see what it does. I constantly remind people that it is God who does the healing and that I am simply a "vehicle" for God's healing power and Grace.

Sometimes, when I give talks, I experience what is biblically referred to as "a word of knowledge." For example, I often have the intuitive sense that that there is a person present with a particular type of pain. This frequently proves to be true. When I lay my hands on people in prayer, I feel heat pass through my hands. I once had to place my hands in water because they got so hot. Sometimes the person seeking healing has an immediate positive response, other times it may be delayed or come in a way that is unexpected. A tremendous peace overcomes the supplicant. Some have reported being so exhausted from this experience that they have gone to bed for several hours.

I am used to people expressing doubt about this ministry. Doubt can be healthy because it often shows that, even with skepticism and doubt, healing can still take place. Interestingly enough, few churches I have come into contact with are openly skeptical about my ministry. In fact, as time goes on, more and more people are referred to the Oratory by health care professionals, including doctors, clergy, psychotherapists and social workers. This obviously reflects a great deal of confidence in the center's healing mission. Such confidence has been further generated through the personal testimonies of those who have been healed through the ministry, of which there are many.

SUGGESTED READING

Simonton, O. Carl, Stephanie Matthews-Simonton, and George Creighton. *Getting Well Again*. New York: Bantam Books, 1980.

NOTE

1. Shamans performed many different roles depending on the tribes they were associated with. Consider some of these diverse roles and their diverse healing practices. Native Americans often believed that illness could be attributed to soul loss (Lyon, 1996, p. 260). It is important to remember, however, that the body may be considered to have several "souls"—the ego soul, the shadow soul, and the dream or free soul (ibid.). A soul may be driven out by some psychic or emotional shock, and in most cases of soul loss the soul travels to the land of the dead (ibid.). In this case, it is the shaman's role to make a journey "toward that realm and fight off hostile forces to bring the soul back to the patient" (ibid.).

When shamans are about to use their healing powers, they have been observed to enter an "ecstatic trance" (ibid., p. 70). In some cultures, this trance is believed to be induced by spirit possession (ibid.). Some shamans may have helping spirits—used when they want to discover something (ibid., p. 89). For example, the Tlingit shaman has several helping spirits, for each of which he has a specially carved mask; when he puts on a mask, the shaman becomes possessed by its spirit, and the words that he speaks are from that spirit (ibid., p. 261).

Animals and plants are also revered for their healing powers. Such animals include the salmon (particularly the coho and early spring salmon), rattlesnake, eagle, woodpecker, wolf, and mountain lion (ibid., pp. 92, 142). Some shamans use the helping spirits of several of these animals (ibid., p. 92). Navaho shamans have apparently claimed that "corn pollen is their most powerful medicine" (ibid., p. 54). Some shamans, referred to as "sucking shamans," use their mouth or some other device to suck the disease or disease object from the sick patient (ibid., p. 55). One shaman from the Oregon seaboard was reported to have sucked out eyes, eggs, lizards, and arrows (ibid., p. 133). For some, it is believed to take 30 years of training before shamans have the ability to cure illness (ibid., p. 140).

SUGGESTED READINGS

Carlson, R., and B. Shield, eds. *Handbook for the Soul*. Boston: Little, Brown, 1995.
Frankl, Viktor E.. *The Doctor and the Soul: An Introduction to Logotherapy*. New York: Alfred A. Knopf, 1957.
Peck, M. Scott. *People of the Lie: The Hope for Healing Human Evil*. New York: Simon & Schuster, 1983.

REFERENCES

The AAUW Report: How Schools Shortchange Girls—A Study of Major Findings on Girls and Education. Washington, DC: AAUW Educational Foundation & National Educational Association, 1992.
Arnold, John D. *Make up Your Mind: The Seven Building Blocks to Better Decisions*. New York: American Management Association, 1978.
Attenborough, Sir Richard. *The Words of Gandhi*. New York: Newmarket Press, 1982.
Banks, Sydney. "Cleaning Out the Clutter." In *Handbook for the Soul*. R. Carlson and B. Shield, eds. Boston: Little, Brown, 1995, pp. 74–77.

Bolen, Jean Shinoda. "Windows of the Soul." In *Handbook for the Soul*. R. Carlson and B. Shield, eds. Boston: Little, Brown, 1995, pp. 3–8.

Borysenko, Joan. "Ensouling Ourselves." In *Handbook for the Soul*. R. Carlson and B. Shield, eds. Boston: Little, Brown, 1995, pp. 45–48.

Boxley, Jeanne, Lynette Lawrance, and Harvey Gruchow. "A Preliminary Study of Eighth Grade Students' Attitudes Toward Rape Myths and Women's Roles." 65 *Journal of School Health* 96–100 (March 1995).

Braillier, Lynn W. "The Suffering of Terminal Illness: Cancer." In *The Hidden Dimension of Illness: Human Suffering*. P.L. Starck and J.P. McGovern, eds. New York: National League for Nursing Press, 1992, pp. 203–25.

Branden, Nathaniel. "Passion and Soulfulness." In *Handbook for the Soul*. R. Carlson and B. Shield, eds. Boston: Little, Brown, 1995, pp. 99–103.

Buber, Martin. *The Way of Man According to the Teachings of Hasidism*. Secaucus, NJ: Citadel Press, 1966.

Bulger, Roger J. "Is Our Society Insensitive to Suffering?" In *The Hidden Dimension of Illness: Human Suffering*. P.L. Starck and J.P. McGovern, eds. New York: National League for Nursing Press, 1992, pp. 53–67.

Cairns, Ed, Liz McWhirter, Ursulla Duffy, et al. "The Stability of Self-Concept in Late Adolescence: Gender and Situational Effects." 11 *Personality and Individual Differences* 937–44 (1990).

Campbell, Don, ed. *Music and Miracles*. Wheaton, IL: Quest Books, 1992.

Cassell, Eric J. "The Nature of Suffering and the Goals of Medicine." 306 *New England Journal of Medicine* 639–45 (1982).

Chirban, John T. "Healing and Spirituality." In *Health and Faith: Medical, Psychological and Religious Dimensions*. Lanham, MD: University Press of America, 1991, pp. 3–11.

Christy, John H. "Prayer as Medicine." 161 *Forbes* 136–40 (March 23, 1998).

Chubb, Nancy H., Carl I. Fertman, and Jennifer L. Ross. "Adolescent Self-Esteem and Locus of Control: A Longitudinal Study of Gender and Age Differences." 32 *Adolescence* 113–29 (Spring 1997).

Courage to Change. New York: Al-Anon Family Group Headquarters, 1992.

Donnelly, Gloria F., and Concetta DeLuca McPeak. "Dreams: Their Function in Health and Illness." 10 *Holistic Nursing Practice* 61–68 (July 1996).

Dossey, Larry. *Healing Words: The Power of Prayer and the Practice of Medicine*. San Francisco: HarperSan Francisco, 1993.

————. *Meaning and Medicine: A Doctor's Tales of Breakthrough and Healing*. New York: Bantam, 1991.

————. *Prayer Is Good Medicine*. New York: HarperCollins, 1996.

Emerson, Ralph Waldo. "Prudence." In *Emerson: Essays and Lectures*. Joel Porte, ed. New York: Library of America, 1983, pp. 357–67.

Frankl, Viktor E. *The Doctor and the Soul: An Introduction to Logotherapy*. New York: Alfred A. Knopf, 1957.

————. "The Significance of Meaning for Health." In *Religion and Medicine: Essays on Meaning, Values, and Health*. D. Belgum, ed. Ames: Iowa State University Press, 1967, pp. 177–85.

————. *The Unconscious God: Psychotherapy and Theology*. New York: Simon & Schuster, 1975.

Fromm, Erich. *The Heart of Man: Its Genius for Good and Evil*. New York: Harper & Row, 1964.

Fulghum, Robert. "Pay Attention." In *Handbook for the Soul*. R. Carlson and B. Shield, eds. Boston: Little, Brown, 1995, pp. 9–17.

Gray, John. "Love Vitamins for Your Soul." In *Handbook for the Soul*. R. Carlson and B. Shield, eds. Boston: Little, Brown, 1995, pp. 54–60.

Harrison, Ruth L. "Spirituality and Hope: Nursing Implications for People with HIV Disease." 12 *Holistic Nursing Practice* 9–16 (Oct. 1997).

Heitman, Elizabeth. "The Influence of Values and Culture in Responses to Suffering." In *The Hidden Dimension of Illness: Human Suffering*. P.L. Starck and J.P. McGovern, eds. New York: National League for Nursing Press, 1992, pp. 81–103.

Hunter, Kathryn Montgomery. *Doctors' Stories: The Narrative Structure of Medical Knowledge*. Princeton, NJ: Princeton University Press, 1991.

Jaret, Peter. "Can Prayer Heal?" 12 *Health* [San Francisco] 48–54 (March 1998).

Jung, Carl. *The Structure and Dynamics of the Psyche*. Collected Works, Vol. VIII. Princeton: Princeton University Press, 1969.

Kabat-Zinn, Jon. *Wherever You Go, There You Are: Mindfulness Meditation in Everyday Life*. New York: Hyperion, 1994.

Kark, Jeremy D., Galia Shemi, Yechiel Friedlander, et al. "Does Religious Observance Promote Health? Mortality in Secular vs. Religious Kibbutzim in Israel." 86 *American Journal of Public Health* 341–46 (March 1996).

Kelsey, Morton. *Healing and Christianity*, 3rd ed. Minneapolis: Augsberg Fortress, 1995.

Kerr, Barbara H. *Smart Girls, Gifted Women*. Dayton: Ohio Psychology Press, 1985.

Koenig, Harold G., Harvey J. Cohen, L.K. George, et al. "Attendance at Religious Services, Interleukin-6, and Other Biological Parameters of Immune Function in Older Adults." 27 *International Journal of Psychiatry & Medicine* 233–50 (1997).

Koenig, Harold G., L.K. George, J.C. Hays, et al. "The Relationship Between Religious Activities and Blood Pressure in Older Adults." 28 *International Journal of Psychiatry & Medicine* 189–213 (1998).

Kushi, Michio, and Edward Esko. *Dream Diagnosis: What Dreams Reveal about Your Health, Relationships, Fortune, and Destiny*. Becket, MA: One Peaceful World, 1996.

Kushner, Harold. "God's Fingerprints on the Soul." In *Handbook for the Soul*. R. Carlson and B. Shield, eds. Boston: Little, Brown, 1995, pp. 18–24.

———. *When Bad Things Happen to Good People*. New York: Schocken Books, 1981.

Langer, Ellen J. *Mindfulness*. Reading, MA: Addison-Wesley, 1989.

Lazare, Aaron. "The Suffering of Shame and Humiliation in Illness." In *The Hidden Dimension of Illness: Human Suffering*. P.L. Starck and J.P. McGovern, eds. New York: National League for Nursing Press, 1992, pp. 227–44.

Lenney, Ellen. "Women's Self-Confidence in Achievement Settings." 84 *Psychological Bulletin* 1–13 (1977).

Levin, Jeffrey S., and Harold Y. Vanderpool. "Is Frequent Religious Attendance Really Conducive to Better Health? Toward an Epidemiology of Religion." 24 *Social Science and Medicine* 589–600 (1989).

Levitan, H. "The Dream in Psychosomatic States." In *The Dream in Clinical Practice*. J.M. Natterson, ed. New York: Aronson, 1980.

Lyon, William S. *Encyclopedia of Native American Healing*. Santa Barbara, CA: ABC-CLIO, 1996.

Manske, Fred A., Jr. *Secrets of Effective Leadership: A Practical Guide to Success*, 2nd ed. Columbia, TN: Leadership Education & Development, 1990.

Martin, John E., and Charles R. Carlson. "Spiritual Dimensions of Health Psychology." In *Behavioral Therapy and Religion*. W.R. Miller and J.E. Martin, eds. Beverly Hills, CA: Sage, 1988, pp. 57–110.

Maslow, Abraham H. *Toward a Psychology of Being*, 2nd ed. Princeton, NJ: D. Van

Nostrand, 1968.

Matthews, Dale A., Anthony L. Suchman, and William T. Branch. "Making 'Connexions': Enhancing the Therapeutic Potential of Patient-Clinical Relationships." 118 *Annals of Internal Medicine* 973–77 (June 15, 1993).

May, Rollo. *The Courage to Create.* New York: W. W. Norton, 1975.

Moore, Thomas. "Embracing the Everyday." In *Handbook for the Soul.* R. Carlson and B. Shield, eds. Boston: Little, Brown, 1995, pp. 25–31.

Moyers, Bill. *Healing and the Mind.* New York: Doubleday, 1993.

Muff, Janet. "From the Wings of Night: Dream Work with Persons Who Have Acquired Immunodeficiency Syndrome." 10 *Holistic Nursing Practice* 69–87 (1996).

Oxman, Thomas E., Daniel H. Freeman, Jr., and Eric D. Manheimer. "Lack of Social Participation or Religious Strength and Comfort as Risk Factors for Death after Cardiac Surgery in the Elderly." 57 *Psychosomatic Medicine* 5–15 (1995).

Pascal, Blaise. *Pensées.* Paris: Didier, 1969.

Peck, M. Scott. *People of the Lie: The Hope for Healing Human Evil.* New York: Simon & Schuster, 1983.

Pipher, Mary. *Reviving Ophelia: Saving the Selves of Adolescent Girls.* New York: Ballantine Books, 1994.

Rogers, Carl. *On Becoming a Person: A Therapist's View of Psychotherapy.* Boston: Houghton Mifflin, 1961.

Sanford, John A. *Healing and Wholeness.* New York: Paulist Press, 1977.

Schweitzer, Albert. *Reverence for Life.* R.H. Fuller, trans. New York: Harper & Row, 1969.

Siegel, Bernie S. *How to Live Between Office Visits: A Guide to Life, Love, and Health.* New York: HarperCollins, 1993.

———. *Love, Medicine and Miracles: Lessons Learned about Self-Healing from a Surgeon's Experience with Exceptional Patients.* New York: Harper & Row, 1986.

Simmons, Roberta G., and Florence Rosenberg. "Sex, Sex Roles, and Self-Image." 4 *Journal of Youth & Adolescence* 229–58 (Sept. 1975).

Sinetar, Marsha. *Living Happily Ever After: Creating Trust, Luck, and Joy.* New York: Villard, 1990.

Starck, Patricia L. "The Management of Suffering in a Nursing Home." In *The Hidden Dimension of Illness: Human Suffering.* P.L. Starck and J.P. McGovern, eds. New York: National League for Nursing Press, 1992, pp. 127–49.

Trecker, J. "Women in U.S. History High School Textbooks." 35 *Social Education* 249–60 (1971).

Tsenam, Khenpo Trosu. "A View from Tibet." In *Oriental Medicine: An Illustrated Guide to the Asian Arts of Healing.* J. Van Alphen and A. Aris, eds. Boston: Shambhala, 1996, pp. 146–53.

Vardey, Lucinda, ed. *God in All Worlds: An Anthology of Contemporary Spiritual Writing.* New York: Pantheon, 1995.

Wallis, Claudia. "Faith and Healing." 147 *Time* 58–64 (June 24, 1996).

Weiss, Brian. "The Soul's Legacy." In *Handbook for the Soul.* R. Carlson and B. Shield, eds. Boston: Little, Brown, 1995, pp. 63–66.

Williams, Walter L. *The Spirit and the Flesh: Sexual Diversity in American Indian Culture.* Boston: Beacon Press, 1986.

Zeller, William W. "Values in Sickness and Health." In *Religion and Medicine: Essays on Meaning, Values and Health.* D. Belgum, ed. Ames: Iowa State University Press, 1967, pp. 256–73.

6

Physician/Patient Communication

INTRODUCTION: THE IMPORTANCE OF COMMUNICATION BETWEEN DOCTOR AND PATIENT

> There are qualities beyond pure medical competence that patients need and
> look for in doctors. They want reassurance. . . . They want to be listened to.
> They want to feel that it makes a difference to the physician, a very big
> difference, whether they live or die. They want to feel that they are in the
> doctor's thoughts. The physician holds the lifeline.
>
> Norman Cousins,
Head First, pp. 308–9

> Given two equally competent physicians, pick the one with a smile and
> optimistic disposition.
>
> Nicholas Wade,
"The Spin Doctors," p. 16.

Doctors relate to patients in different ways. Because they generally have superior medical knowledge to patients, some prefer to make decisions for patients or, at least, share little of their "power" in the doctor/patient relationship. Others prefer a more "equal" doctor/patient relationship in which decision making is shared. The former type of relationship has typically been called "paternalistic," the latter more egalitarian.

The paternalistic relationship, in which the doctor makes decisions without imput from the patient, is still more common (Roter & Hall, 1993, p. 25). This type of relationship is preferred by the elderly and those with low incomes and social status (ibid.). Only 8 percent of physicians have indicated that they have accommodated patients' demands for decision-making power (ibid., p. 30).

Within the past 20 years, however, there has been some erosion of the paternalistic doctor/patient relationship. The changed "power differential" in such a relationship has probably resulted from patient efforts to seek an egalitarian relationship, which has allowed them to engage in more negotiation with doctors over what is important and what should be done (see Quill, 1983).

Doctors advocating for patient-centered medicine have respected patients' desires for a greater role in decision making (Stewart, Brown, Weston, et al., 1995). However, a patients' rights movement has probably made patients more consumer-oriented and, therefore, more aggressive in requesting a larger say in matters affecting their health.

Patient efforts to have greater control in the doctor/patient relationship are illustrated by the fact that half of the public reports having challenged their doctors (Haug & Lavin, 1983). Some doctors place the patient at the center of the doctor/patient relationship and solicit the patient's feedback on issues such as the type of treatments preferred—it is noteworthy that 69 percent of patients in one study of those with breast cancer preferred to participate in treatment-related decisions (Blanchard, Labrecque, Ruckdeschel, et al., 1988); these types of physicians are rated as more competent by their peers (Hall & Roter, 1988).

No matter what style of relationship doctors have with their patients, there is currently much emphasis on the way in which doctors talk to patients (Roter & Hall, 1993). As discussed in chapter 2, the words a doctor uses have the powerful ability to heal or harm. Studies have shown that the capacity of the doctor to enhance the patient's ability to remain healthy may depend upon factors such as the doctor's ability to provide encouragement, hope, and optimism. For example, although 64 percent of patients who received good news from their doctor in one study (because they were told that they could expect to improve in a few days) did better; only 39 percent of patients who had a "negative encounter" with this same physician did better (Thomas, 1987).

Some studies also suggest that treating patients with compassion has measurable outcomes and effects on health. In one study, patients who met with anesthesiologists before scheduled surgery and who were paid "warm and sympathetic" attention, were discharged 2.7 days before patients who were not paid such attention (Egbert, Battit, Welch, et al., 1964). In a randomized trial of compassionate versus "authoritarian" approaches to the homeless in an emergency department, sympathetic care reduced repeat visits (Redelmeier, Molin, & Tibshirani, 1995).

Knowing how to communicate effectively with patients may require the doctor to learn to focus on patients and to understand their many questions and concerns. As discussed in chapter 3, to treat patients compassionately and effectively, doctors must understand the patients' need to be heard; ways in which discrimination and stigma undermine patients' will to live; ways in which the physical limitations of illness may render patients less productive and jeopardize their self-esteem; the extent of support patients have; the nature of patients' fears; the culture and community with which patients identify; the factors patients use to decide whether to undergo or refuse medications or treatments; and patients' beliefs and expectations regarding health care.

THE BREAKDOWN IN COMMUNICATION
BETWEEN DOCTOR AND PATIENT

There has been a significant breakdown in physician/patient communication over the past few decades. The increase in medical malpractice lawsuits, often due to patients' disapproval of their doctors' style, and the fact that patients increasingly change their doctors are indications of this breakdown.

Documentation of this change has come from patients themselves. In a poll of 1500 patients, 85 percent had changed physicians in the last five years or were thinking of changing physicians because of the doctor's style or office manner (Cousins, 1989, p. 32). These patients were troubled by physician insensitivity to their needs, poor communication techniques, lack of respect for patient views, and an overemphasis on technology. In a meta-analysis of patient satisfaction surveys (see Chart 6-1), patients were least satisfied with physician informativeness, medical care cost, the wait at the doctor's office, and the physician's inattentiveness to psychosocial problems (Hall & Dornan, 1988).

Chart 6-1
Levels of Patient Satisfaction with Their Doctors

Most Satisfied with   *Moderately Satisfied with*

Doctor's humaneness   Facilities
Technical competence   Continuity of care
Outcome of care   Access to Care

Least Satisfied with

Doctor's Informativeness
Medical Care Cost
Wait at office
Attentiveness to psychosocial problems

Physician Insensitivity

Physician insensitivity may obviously take many forms but certainly includes behavior such as the following:

- Repeatedly reminding patients with terminal illnesses that their diseases are fatal: One woman with AIDS, for example, was reminded by her doctor at each office visit that AIDS was "uniformly fatal," and, therefore, she must follow her treatment to the letter (Dossey, 1993, p. 140). This patient reported feeling depressed after every office visit and felt her doctor's emotional attitude was killing her (ibid., pp. 140–41).

- A reminder that there is "nothing more" that the doctor can do for the patient: Although doctors may be frustrated that there are no new medicines or technology to alleviate their patients' symptoms, they must be more sensitive to their ability to support patients and to offer them hope.
- Ray, who had been in and out of the hospital several times with cancer, had asked his doctor when he would be able to leave. The doctor answered, "Oh, I don't think you'll make it this time." Ray reportedly died within minutes (Siegel, 1986, p. 39).

Poor Communication Techniques

Among the main reasons that patients remain critical of the office manner or "style" of their doctors are that these doctors

- are not open-minded and do not encourage or invite questions from patients: Dr. Bernie S. Siegel has suggested that "[o]pen-mindedness is the hallmark of all physicians who are truly interested in helping their patients" (ibid., p. 37).
- do not offer patients any hope: This includes frequent reference to the fact that "nothing more can be done" or reminders that illnesses are terminal.
- quote statistics (often on rates of recovery) without keeping them in perspective: Although it is reasonable for doctors to refer to probabilities and risks when patients seek to know their prognosis, they must be cautious to remind patients that not everyone falls within the mean or the median. When death is a possible prognosis, doctors should also note that no doctor can really predict when another will die.

Open-minded physicians would be prepared to acknowledge that patients may have very effective solutions for their problems—particularly with regard to their psychosocial problems. But, as discussed later, even when a physical illness is involved, physicians should be prepared to accept the fact that patients' goals for therapy and/or treatment may be different from what physicians might recommend. Doctors who might be uncomfortable with or disagree with a patient's ideas should consider such disagreements as opportunities to create win-win situations, "where the ideas of both may lead to a more creative solution" (Stewart, Brown, Weston, et al., 1995, p. 134). Then the doctor/patient relationship can take on the characteristics of a partnership.

Lack of Respect for Patient Views

Fear of being humiliated by their doctor is the most common reason patients give for not asking their doctor questions (Tuckett, Boulton, & Williams, 1985). But even if patients felt comfortable asking their doctor questions, doctors frequently interrupt patients—on average 18 seconds into the patient's description of the presenting problem (Frankel & Beckman, 1989). This precludes any real understanding of the patient's physical problem.

Some doctors have suggested some of the following ways to respect the patient's views. Dr. Eric Cassell has said that doctors must defer to solutions that, from the patient's point of view, would be adequate (Cassell, 1985). Some patients prefer to be treated in the least invasive manner possible (see Stewart, Brown, Weston, et al., 1995, p. 65). A woman with metastatic breast disease may only want treatment for the control of her symptoms (such as pain management) rather than treatment to slow the progression of her disease (ibid., p. 64).

Overemphasis on Technology

> [Good physicians] do not lose sight of the lives out of which patients' choices come and into which medical therapy must intrude.
>
> Kathryn Montgomery Hunter,
> *Doctors' Stories*, pp. 158–59

The corporate invasion of the health care industry (see Starr, 1982, pp. 429 et seq.) has made health care a business that must be profitable. The emphasis on profitability means that many tests will be done (because hospitals make money from tests). Oddly enough, however, the increased prevalence of technological approaches to aid in diagnosis may not always promote health. For example, because there are too many mammography machines each is underutilized. This doubles the cost of each test. Because many cannot afford the test, we have too little breast cancer screening (Schiff, Bindman, Brennan, et al., 1994).

The emphasis on profitability also means that more patients must be seen (consequently, doctors can spend less time with patients). Even in 1988, before widespread patient enrollment in health maintenance organizations, doctors in family practice spent an average of 14 minutes with a patient during a medical visit and doctors in internal medicine 19 minutes with a patient (Nelson & McLemore, 1988).

The increased use of technology is believed to be a major reason that patients are seen as "objects." One astute physician has noted, "[w]hile seeing more, we are often at high risk of hearing less" (Jackson, 1992, p. 1630). For valid reasons, doctors focus on "objective evidence" because the main reason most people seek their services is the treatment of physical illness. But if patients were to read their medical charts, many would be surprised by how little evidence the medical record contained about psychosocial issues—they would think, "This is not really me!"[1] For this reason, some doctors have suggested that in order to "humanize" the medical record or the presentation of the medical "case," physicians add a sentence or two describing "the patient's understanding of the illness and how the illness [is] affecting the patient's life" (Hunter, 1991, p. 168).[2]

Technology may enable doctors to prolong patients' lives, but it may not ensure that patients have any appreciable quality of life. There is much to be said for living a better as opposed to a longer life. With the overemphasis on technology doctors may not even come to view death as natural—simply because technology can delay death. Consider the following account, written by a physician describing an experience during his internship in which he "assaulted a desperately ill patient with the awesome power of technology before he finally realized the need to let his patient die in peace" (Weinberg, 1988).

I was called to the emergency room on a cold winter evening to admit a 76-year-old man complaining of dyspnea (shortness of breath). I examined my new patient, his X-rays and his sputum: a simple case of pneumococcal pneumonia. I took cultures, started an IV, wrote orders for antibiotics, and as my patient was wheeled off to the wards, I went to talk to his wife, who waited outside.

"He has pneumonia," I explained, "but the germ is very sensitive to antibiotics. He'll need to stay with us a few days, but then he should be as good as new."

"We've been married over 50 years, Doctor," she said.

"How nice."

"He's an old man, Doctor," she said in a way that seemed more like a warning than a statement.

My new patient, however, did not do well. Once on the ward, he rapidly slipped into respiratory failure. . . .

I moved my patient to the intensive care unit and intubated him. But his oxygenation remained poor, and he developed signs of congestive heart failure.

An hour later, I was summoned urgently back to the intensive care unit. My patient's blood pressure had suddenly dropped and he was now cyanotic (bluish or purplish discoloration of skin due to a lack of oxygen in the blood). A quick physical exam revealed a pneumothorax on the left side. . . .

As my patient's blood pressure fell even further, I returned to the waiting room to speak to his wife. . . . But before I could finish, the woman interrupted me:

"I've been coming to this hospital long enough to know that you're a good doctor, and that you have done what you could," she said. "But now it's his time."

I returned to the intensive care unit, faced the bed in which my patient lay, and was suddenly overcome with a sense of horror. In four short hours I had presided over the transmogrification of a human being into a jumbled mass of tubes, wires and tape, and in the process had ripped him away from his source of love and comfort. Instead of a brilliant man of medicine, I now saw myself as an insensitive torturer unable to recognize the simple fact that this man was beyond my help. I took the order book and undid what I could (the doctor noted that he wrote such things as "Do Not Resuscitate," "Discontinue arterial catheter and restraints.").

[After the patient died, the elderly woman left the intensive care unit and placed her arm on the doctor's arm.]

"Thank you, Doctor."

"But . . . he died," I blurted out.

"Yes, but he died peacefully."

Inattentiveness to Psychosocial Problems

Patients' psychosocial problems typically involve their ability to adapt to social and environmental changes and the physical limitations imposed by illness. One study has indicated that 80 percent of patients' social problems are not known to physicians (Stewart & Buck, 1977). As already discussed in chapter 2, doctors discuss psychosocial problems much less with the elderly than with their younger patients (Roter & Hall, 1993, p. 41).

Patients need to be able to share their emotional pain with their doctors, even doctors who are not psychiatrists. Often sharing their pain allows it to be transformed (see Siegel, 1993, p. 142). One orthopedic surgeon in Viet Nam, for example, cared for a soldier who fractured his leg in a helicopter crash in which he was the sole survivor (ibid.). Because the patient complained of continued pain, the doctors changed and rechanged his cast. However, after the patient talked about his survivor's guilt, his pain went away.

Chapter 8 suggests an expanded role for physicians that would enable them to be more sensitive to patients' psychosocial problems. This suggested expanded role includes some of the following:

- Taking more time to know patients and their families so that doctors can understand more fully how patients are adapting to their illnesses.
- Learning how patients' families have adapted to their illness and whether they are being appropriately supportive.
- Counseling patients who are depressed and dissatisfied with their jobs.
- Encouraging patients and bolstering their will to live: This may involve helping them determine what is important in their lives and may provide them with meaning.
- Attempting to find the cause of patients' depression—rather than just treating the symptoms of depression with medication: By helping patients identify the cause of their depression, doctors may not only begin to help patients identify the steps to be taken that may gradually eliminate the depression but may assist them to regain control of their lives. A pill for depression may mask the depression but may not provide the solution for having a better or rich life.

IMPROVING COMMUNICATION BETWEEN DOCTOR AND PATIENT

One critical mechanism to repair physician/patient communication is for doctors to refocus on the patient and to

- resist efforts to judge or dismiss patient concerns and questions and allow patients to express their range of feelings.
- appreciate the limitations drugs and therapies may cause—and how these limitations affect the patient's life.
- show compassion by carefully listening to patient concerns and expectations.
- avoid imposing their ethical biases upon patients.
- allow patients to maintain hope.

Resisting Efforts to Judge or Dismiss Patient Concerns

Patients do not consider it respectful when physicians minimize their concerns. Although patients are usually satisfied with the technical quality of their care, they often report that their "personal and subjective needs have often been unmet" (Gerteis, Edgman-Levitan, Daley, et al., 1993). Others note that patients tend to be satisfied if they believe that someone has paid attention to their concerns (Brown, Nelson, Bronkesh, et al., 1993; Oxler, 1997). In short, failure to listen to or provide an appropriate response to the patient is failure to perceive the patient as having something worthy to say and is likely to affect the trust needed for a good doctor/patient relationship (Oxler, 1997).

Bernie S. Siegel has said that it is the doctor's role to accept patients and try to help them (Siegel, 1986, p. 53), regardless of whether physicians agree with the patients' decisions. For example, oncologists may feel that patients should accept the toxic effects of radiation and chemotherapy over the short term in order to have a chance at a longer life—which may include the possibility of remission from cancer. Patients, however, may prefer to focus on the quality of life they have and forgo treatment, even though it may mean a shortened life expectancy.

Doctors should not dismiss a patient's concerns merely because they do not have answers. Oliver Sacks, the British neurologist and author of *Awakenings*, *The Man Who Mistook His Wife for a Hat*, and *A Leg to Stand On*, described his encounters with various physicians after sustaining a leg injury in which he subsequently lost all sensation in his leg. When Sacks complained that his leg did not work, his doctor said that there was "nothing to worry about" (Sacks, 1984, p. 105). After Sacks accused his doctor of not listening to him, the doctor responded that he couldn't "waste his time with experiences like this" (ibid., p. 107).

The interview with Susan Connor at the end of this chapter, reveals that, for years, some health care professionals dismissed a mother's allegation that there was something wrong with her son. This case story would seem to suggest that doctors who do not know what is wrong with a patient are obliged to make an appropriate referral to physicians who may be more knowledgeable about certain conditions.

Doctors should allow patients to express many of their feelings, including their anger, without being ready either to dismiss the patient's feelings or to respond with anger. Many writers about issues in mind/body medicine have noted the relationship between long-term survivors and their physicians—including their ability to disagree with or express anger toward their physicians (Siegel, 1986, p. 25; Rabkin, Remien, Katoff, et al., 1993). Michael Callen, a long-term AIDS survivor, has noted that such survivors often have an "extraordinary relationship" with their health care provider (Callen, 1990, p. 45). He has stressed the need for patients to be skeptical of new treatments (ibid., p. 194) because "[s]cientific or medical truth cannot be determined in a democratic fashion" (ibid., p. 195).

Doctors rate about 15 percent of their patients as "difficult" (Sharp, 1998) and they have described their relationship with such patients as "poor" (see Siegel, 1986, p. 25). But being "difficult" is a matter of perspective—behavior one physician might consider "being difficult" might not be viewed in the same way by another. Doctors who characterize their patients as difficult are also likely to be so characterized by their patients.

Some have said that it is irresponsible for physicians to separate themselves from patients who disagree with them (Cousins, 1983, p. 255). Other physicians, however, have admitted to screening patients on the basis of whether they feel some rapport with them (see Janiger & Goldberg, 1993, p. 56). As patients demand more information or decision making in matters that affect their health, a certain paradigm shift is occurring in the medical profession—a shift in which the focus is on the patient's wishes and not necessarily those of the doctor. As already suggested, this paradigm shift views the doctor as a counselor, partner, and facilitator (see Hawkins, 1993, p. 130).

Appreciating the Limitations of Drugs and Therapies

Human beings have tremendous needs to be productive, to benefit their immediate families, acquire status, be recognized, or benefit their society. Remaining productive maintains our self-esteem. Consequently, the limitations imposed by medications or surgery, by jeopardizing people's abilities to be productive, can significantly affect their capacity to maintain feelings of competence and self-worth. Physicians need to be particularly sensitive to the type of limitations that drugs or therapies may impose upon patients.

Consider these examples of limitations that either drugs or treatments imposed upon patients and how, in their view, such therapies jeopardized their quality of life. What is particularly shocking about the following scenarios is that there is no explicit evidence that doctors were particularly sensitive to the limitations these therapies imposed upon their patients.

- Elizabeth, a woman with breast cancer who had a mastectomy and lymph node dissection that removed 18 lymph nodes from her armpit, focused on the limitations imposed by the lymphedema she experienced after surgery, which caused the swelling of her arm (Warren, 1996, pp. 13 et seq.). Elizabeth is a physical fitness trainer who lifted weights and who did not expect that her surgery would dramatically affect her ability to work. Her physician never informed her before the dissection that her arm would no longer be able to tolerate heavy weights (ibid., p. 22). Elizabeth expected her doctor to have discussed the pros and cons of lymph node dissection and the likelihood that she would experience lymphedema.
- Kay is manic-depressive and a science researcher at Johns Hopkins who studies this inherited illness. Her illness is managed with lithium although she still experiences "inevitable swings of mood and energy" (Jamison, 1995, p. 213). Kay herself, not her treating psychiatrist, reduced the amount of lithium she took (ibid., p. 167). She reported that the lower dose allowed her to handle stress better (and enhanced her productivity), gave her a "clarity of thinking," and brought a "vividness and intensity of experience" back into her life (ibid.). It was only through her own initiative that she was able to improve the quality of her life by adjusting her medication levels.

The Compassionate Physician: Learning to Care for the Patient

Not every patient can be saved, but his illness may be eased by the way the doctor responds to him—and in responding to him the doctor may save himself. . . . It may be necessary to give up some of his authority in exchange for his humanity, but as the old family doctors knew, this is not a bad bargain. In learning to talk to his patients, the doctor may talk himself back into loving his work. He has little to lose and everything to gain by letting the sick man into his heart.

Anatole Broyard,
Intoxicated by My Illness, p. 57

It is much more important to know what sort of patient has a disease than to know what sort of disease a patient has.

Sir William Osler
quoted in Cousins,
The Healing Heart, p. 256

One must pick one's situations, and adjust the truth to the judgment of wise kindness.

Hans Zinsser,
As I Remember Him, p. 142

As Osler suggests, it is critical for doctors to focus on the whole person, not just disease. When doctors learn the patient's story, they are able to understand their patients' views of the world and of their illnesses. Sometimes patients just cry out to be understood. To understand, doctors must be able to listen to patients.

Compassionate physicians are those who have learned how to care for patients. *Caring* has been defined as helping others grow and actualize themselves and achieve their human potential (Watson, 1988).

Patients know when their doctors seem concerned whether they live or die; concerned enough to take extra measures to ensure their well-being, such as an occasional house call; or concerned enough to reach out to the patient's family and provide appropriate information to enhance their capacity to care for them.

Physicians focus on the whole person when they

- listen to patients and allow them to tell their stories, how they react to their illnesses, how they are coping with them, how their illnesses have affected their daily lives—and even their goals and dreams.
- ask questions about the patient's family, for it is possible that if one family member is in distress, the entire family may be under stress.
- ask whether patients face any particular discrimination: The worries caused by palpable discrimination often directly affect the patient's health. For example, people with AIDS may have been abandoned by their families, fired from their jobs, or denied coverage by their insurance carriers. People with hemophilia are often the victims of discrimination—particularly by insurance companies who seek to limit the payment for factor VIII.

Listening has risen to the level of an art because it is so rare. But listening to another is one of the best ways to show respect. Listening is respectful because it provides the opportunity for the other to be acknowledged and, as noted later, to be understood.

Our egos cause us to focus on the next thing we are going to say—and this is one main reason that listening is so rare. We often do not take the time to hear what another has to say because we are so quick to judge, evaluate, or critique their ideas or positions.

Compassion also stems from a genuine desire to understand the patient. Listening is only one way in which doctors can come to understand patients. Another, more powerful, way stems from caring about them. This quality comes from the interior world (e.g., personality and spirituality) of the doctor.

Compassionate physicians focus on their patients' needs, not on themselves. Compassion emanates from understanding patients' circumstances and appreciating the factors that may contributed to their illnesses, an appreciation that patients are more than the diseases they have.

It may not be easy work to understand the patient and to view the world from the patient's perspective. Doctors genuinely interested in understanding their patients might heed the words of Confucius: "To know that we know what we know, and that we do not know what we do not know, that is true knowledge" (Sayre, 1985).[3]

To understand the patient's world better, doctors could ask about the activities that are important to patients and how patients structure their days to be able to accomplish those activities. Because illness may interrupt patients' abilities to engage in daily activities, doctors who understand what is important to patients have a clear understanding of what provides meaning to them.

Chapter 1 noted a range of circumstances affecting patients' health—from their environment, to the amount of support they may have at home and in their community, to whether they have financial concerns or are subject to discrimination. Consequently, the compassionate physician seeks to understand what the person—not just the person with the disease—is going through, experiencing, or feeling. The compassionate physician attempts to understand how particular patients suffer from their disease (see the discussion in chapter 5), how their disease affects their ability to find meaning in their lives, and how their degree of happiness (or sadness or depression) is affected.

Many physicians have been trained to be "detached" and to hide their concern and compassion because they assume that this is part of being professional and that is what patients expect of them (Fallowfield, 1993, p. 477). When physicians hide their concern and compassion, patients feel they are being unsympathetic, but physicians often do not recognize this effect of their "clinical detachment." Such detachment may undermine the trust and confidence in the physician so necessary for the proper formation of a physician/patient relationship. And as already mentioned, patients' will to live is bolstered by physicians who genuinely show concern about whether they live or die.

But one physician who treats people with HIV/AIDS addresses the appropriateness of physicians' involvement in their patients' lives and, perhaps, even the development of personal relationships with them. He noted that he has surrounded himself "with the afflicted, the [HIV] infected, the affected, and their caretakers—my patients and colleagues, my peers, my friends, and, ultimately my family. And I am faced tonight with the ironic, wonderful, and awful realization that there is no greater joy than that which comes from caring for someone in need" (Cohan, 1996, p. 47). Earlier in his essay, Dr. Cohan admits: "[s]uffice it to say that Phil and I broke a few rules. In fact, we reinvented them. We discovered that a close loving friendship and a concurrent doctor/patient relationship were not destructive or even mutually exclusive." Such a relationship obviously allows the doctor to see the patient as a whole person. These sentiments, however, are quite contrary to much medical advice to remain "detached" from the patient.

There are many reasons why it may be difficult for physicians to show their concern for patients. First, the physician may seek to be "detached" so as not to be overwhelmed by the patient's suffering (Siegel, 1989, p. 130). Many studies discuss the difficulty doctors often have relating to their sickest patients. One study concluded that physicians liked their healthier patients more than their less healthy patients, even when standard sociodemographic characteristics were controlled (Hall, Epstein, DeCiantis, et al., 1993). Second, physicians may feel inadequate in treating patients because "modern medicine" provides no acceptable treatment. Doctors may unnecessarily consider themselves "failures" if they cannot help or cure patients. And, at least for medical students, death is viewed as a failure (Olin, 1972). Doctors do not fully understand that many patients only expect a doctor's care (e.g., treatment), not necessarily a cure (Siegel, 1989, p. 149).

Compassion is also shown by involvement, not detachment. Involvement includes attempts to

- engage patients in conversation.
- respect a patient's views.
- become involved (or at least interested) in the patient's life—knowing about the patient's interests and family.

Allowing Patients to Maintain Hope

For a patient to be told that two out of every five persons with a certain illness do not last out the year is not as motivating as to be told that three out of five patients do survive their ordeal.

Norman Cousins,
The Healing Heart, pp. 135–36

The purposes of effective physician/patient communication, however, are, as Norman Cousins has suggested, to give the patient a lifeline—and, as Bernie

Siegel suggests, "to help the patient find an inner reason for living" (Siegel, 1986, p. 97). This "lifeline" is often described as giving patients hope, while telling them the truth (Brody, 1961).

Norman Cousins and Bernie Siegel have both cautioned the medical profession to tread carefully in giving a poor prognosis to a patient—because words may deprive the patient of hope and the healing power associated with hope. This admonition must be viewed in light of evidence that people who expect to die within a certain period often do (Cousins, 1989, p. 98) ("People move along the path of their expectations"). In other words, patients who receive "negative information" may give up hope.

Cousins, Frankl, and Siegel all seem to suggest that the physician's obligation is to give patients hope:

- Giving them reassurance: Some have said that doctors can bolster the confidence of their patients such that they can get well (Pelletier, 1977, p. 272). The substantial correlation between hope and survival is of course related to studies that link optimism and survival (Kaplan & Camacho, 1983) and those that link happiness and longevity (Wolf, 1959).
- Allowing the patient to focus on future goals: Bernie Siegel defines hope as "seeing that the outcome you want is possible, and then working for it" (Siegel, 1986, p. 178).
- Counseling patients that not everyone falls "within the mean": According to Norman Cousins, "[n]o more important lesson can be learned by medical students than that no one knows enough to make a pronouncement of doom" (Cousins, 1989, p. 98). For example, some patients may be outliers—those on the periphery of the bell curve who are way beyond the mean. However, outliers are often disregarded in scientific calculations as a "necessary precaution" (Hirshberg & Barasch, 1995, p. 288).
- Remaining aware that a patient's belief in treatment, even though the treatment may be ineffective, may be keeping the patient alive.[4]

Physicians must also be cautious about giving "negative information" to persons in certain cultural groups, such as Native Americans. As discussed in chapter 2, traditionally Native Americans and some Asians believe that talking about "bad news" may bring about its occurrence (Carrese & Rhodes, 1995). On the other hand, different ethnic groups will want "negative" information. Puerto Ricans may prefer to be informed of their terminal illness in order to "complete their relationship" with particular friends or relatives such as saying something that has been left unsaid (Harwood, 1981, p. 167).

Refusing to Impose Ethical Views upon the Patient

Physicians should not impose their ethical views. Suppose patients with a variety of inherited disorders seek to have children, even though the children may be born with the genetic condition inherited from one of the parents. It is quite possible that a physician would oppose the couple's having children under such circumstances.

Although doctors have a legal duty to inform parents with genetic defects (or even carrying recessive genes for certain defects) that they may have a child with the defect, whether it be manic-depressive illness, mental retardation, Tay- Sachs disease, or hemophilia, doctors should refrain from making value judgments as to the potential "worth" of a child with a genetic defect. This area, is, of course, fraught with a great deal of ethical complexity, and the "best advice" is difficult to come by, particularly in light of the facts that some inherited conditions are more treatable than others, some are fatal within a short time after birth, and for parents unable to bear the economic costs of treating such conditions, society may have an economic interest in determining whether some children will live or die.

In *An Unquiet Mind: A Memoir of Moods and Madness*, Kay Redfield Jamison, a scientist studying and a person with manic-depressive illness, notes a "cruel" encounter with a physician who thought that she should not have children and that she would be an incompetent mother solely because of her manic-depressive illness—of note is the fact that her illness was substantially controlled by taking lithium (Jamison, 1995, p. 191). Jamison argues that "[e]ven in my blackest depressions, I never regretted having been born. [Although] I had wanted to die, . . . that is peculiarly different from regretting having been born" (ibid.).

Respecting the Coping Mechanisms of a Patient

[A] young doctor developed a melanosarcoma, and correctly diagnosed the disease himself. His colleagues vainly tried to convince him that there was no sarcoma. They went so far as to deceive him, showing him negative urine reactions—after exchanging his urine for someone else's. The young doctor stole into the laboratory at night and himself conducted a urine test. As the disease progressed, his friends feared that he would attempt suicide. But instead the young doctor began increasingly to doubt his original correct diagnosis. When metastases of the liver had already set in, he began diagnosing the symptoms as those of a harmless liver affliction. Thus he unconsciously deceived himself—because in the last stages of the disease the will to live was rebelling against impending death. We must respect this will to live—not deny a man the right to life for the sake of some ideology.

Viktor E. Frankl,
The Doctor and the Soul, pp. 54–55

In dealing with a terminally ill patient, Frankl cautions the medical profession not to be too quick to confront or pierce the patient's denial system. For many, denial is a critical coping mechanism that enables them to continue to live their lives without having to admit to themselves that their death is imminent.

Communication with and Respecting the Needs of the Dying Patient

Where persons die in hospitals, as opposed to hospices, there is every reason to believe that staff efforts at sympathetic communication are ineffective. In one study of inpatients known to be dying, staff gave greater priority to taking the patient's blood pressure and pulse rate than to relieving the patient's pain (Mills, Davies, & Macrae, 1994).

What is particularly shocking to a first-time reader about the medical profession's treatment of the terminally ill is that pain is undertreated (Rich, 1997; Shapiro, 1996). Despite the fact that patients remain concerned about the alleviation of pain at the end-of-life, experts agree that the terminally ill in nursing homes, hospitals, and those who die at home are undertreated for pain (Rutchick, 1999; Stolberg, 1998a). More than one-quarter of nursing home residents who complain of pain are given nothing for their pain, not even aspirin (Stolberg, 1998c). Although hospice emphasizes pain management, in some states it is difficult to qualify for entering hospice.

Some of the main barriers patients face in being adequately treated for pain are the following:

- Doctors can be disciplined for overprescribing: but patients in some states are filing complaints before state medical boards for a physician's failure to prescribe powerful narcotics to treat a patient's pain (Stolberg, 1998a).
- Medical schools and residency training programs fail to teach doctors how to care for people at the end of life (Miller, 1998).
- Doctors often have irrational beliefs regarding addiction to painkillers (Gallagher, 1997).
- Overbearing actions of regulatory authorities chills the legitimate prescription practices of physicians; one case noted that physicians avoid treating pain patients in order to avoid prosecution (*Hoover v. Agency for Health Care Administration*, 1996).

The poor state of end-of-life care (often called *palliative care*) in the United States might have sustained the movement for assisted suicide and has undoubtedly contributed to the growth of the hospice movement (20 percent of persons who die in the United States do so in hospices) (Stolberg, 1998b). For a family member's perspective about the contributions of hospice to more humane care, see the interview with Karin Schneider at the end of this chapter.

CHAPTER SUMMARY

Although doctors have different communication styles with patients, there are two typical forms of the doctor/patient relationship—the paternalistic relationship in which the doctor retains a great deal of the "power," and hence, decision making in the relationship, and the more egalitarian relationship, in which decision making is shared and the doctor frequently becomes the patient's adviser. The patients' rights movement over the past 20 years, and the current focus upon patient-centered medicine, are bringing prominence to this latter model.

Over the past few decades patients have reported being troubled by physician insensitivity to their needs, poor communication techniques, lack of respect for patient views, overemphasis on technology, and inattentiveness to their psychosocial needs. Insensitive physicians may typically remind patients that their illnesses are fatal or that there is "nothing more that can be done." Because such physicians either discourage or irritate patients, it is not surprising that patients seek other physicians for their care.

Poor communication techniques are another reason for patients to be dissatisfied with their care. Patients often expect their physicians to be open-minded and encourage them to ask questions. And physicians must be willing to hear the patient's answer; consequently, physicians must be careful not to interrupt. Many patients also expect their doctors to continue to offer them hope. Physicians can give patients hope in such ways as reassuring them to allow them to focus on future goals; counseling them that not everyone falls "within the mean"; and remaining sensitive to the extent to which a patient believes in a treatment—even if the doctor considers it worthless.

A lack of respect for patient views is also a barrier to effective care and treatment. The most common reason patients give for not asking their doctor questions is the fear of being humiliated. Doctors must recognize that they may disagree with or be uncomfortable with the reasons for a patient's decisions; such disagreements could be opportunities for doctors to create "win-win" situations, in which the ideas of both parties may be used to craft more creative solutions.

An overemphasis on technology is a major reason why patients feel they are perceived as "objects." Doctors must allow patients to feel that they are concerned whether they live or die—and that they are more interested in how patients, and not just their diseases, are doing.

Physicians' inattentiveness to patients' psychosocial problems troubles patients. One study indicates that 80 percent of patients' social problems are unknown to their physicians. Unless physicians understand their patients' worlds, patients may feel that their physicians do not really care about them.

It is important to make a distinction between the art of medicine and the science of medicine. The art of medicine involves compassionately listening to and understanding the patient, whereas the practice of the science of medicine implies technical competence. Expertise in the practice of one of these components does not necessarily mean expertise in the practice of the other.

It is also debatable whether physicians can remain "detached" yet compassionate. Physicians may remain detached because they fear being overwhelmed by a patient's suffering or because they consider themselves failures if they cannot offer patients a cure. Doctors must realize, however, that patients often expect only care, not necessarily a cure.

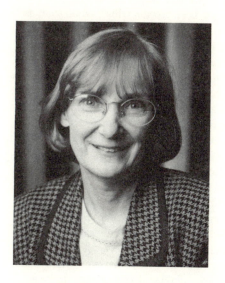

AN INTERVIEW WITH SUSAN CONNOR

I'm a law professor at a Chicago-area law school. I'd like to tell you about my experiences with the medical establishment (and an unsympathetic school system) in my efforts to help my son David, now 16 years old, who was an unhappy child for most of his 16 years. After eight years searching for an explanation (and treatment) for my son's unhappiness, a pediatric neurologist was able to solve our family problem.

I had the first inklings that something was wrong with my son when he was in pre-school and was five years old. He seemed to be overwhelmed by his day at school and practically sat in a trance in an effort to "regroup." By the time David was in the first grade, I noticed that he never invited friends to our home nor was he often invited to people's homes. Because he seemed so unhappy, I spoke with my pediatrician about him. He said that my son would grow out of it.

When David's unhappiness continued, I thought he was allergic to foods. After a battery of tests costing $1,200 and confirming that David had many allergies, no concrete recommendations were made. I even approached the social worker at David's public school to see if my son could be evaluated for emotional problems. I was told that even if I requested an evaluation under the law protecting "disabled" children, it would be a year before any such evaluation would take place.

I then took David to a private psychologist. David thought there was nothing wrong with himself. He clearly did not want to see this doctor and, as a result, he attempted to run away from home. David stopped seeing this psychologist.

We returned to our pediatrician's group practice and saw a different pediatrician from the one we had previously seen. Again, this pediatrician felt there was nothing physically wrong with David and that any psychological approach to the problem was inappropriate unless David were "deranged."

We then found a different psychologist who David saw for five years (when he was in grades 3–7). We paid this psychologist $120/hour and he stonewalled any referral to a psychiatrist because the psychiatrist might use medications to treat David's condition. This psychologist, the graduate of a prestigious institution, said that although David was depressed, the use of anti depressants would be inappropriate because they would thwart David's emotional development (note: this view was challenged by other physicians we were to consult).

Around this time, my spouse and I decided it was best to send David to a private school because his academic performance had deteriorated. He was typically getting D's in courses. He showed me lists of assignments which he had not done and sometimes there were 20 items on the list. Because the tuition at this school was $14,000/year, we decided to have David's therapist meet his teacher to see what could be done to help David. The therapist thought that David needed compassionate human contact and suggested that while addressing David, the teacher could put her hand on his shoulder. Even though the teacher had 10 students in her class, she would not make these attempts.

By the time David was in the seventh grade, we took him to a general internist who seemed to dismiss our concerns about our son—noting that he was "just a teenager." Close to this time, I coincidentally met a clinical psychologist who was on contract to my daughter's school district. This psychologist referred us to a pediatric neurologist. After a battery of tests, he determined that David's brain serotonin levels were abnormally high. He explained that excess serotonin caused overstimulation in the brain—apparently the synapses in the brain are stimulated at such a rapid rate that a child actually "shuts down" because he cannot process all the information his brain is receiving. To combat this problem, David was prescribed 20 mg of Aventyl (a drug used to treat depression but at doses of 200 mg) and Paxil, a drug to control David's frequent temper tantrums—which had occurred several times a day.

With these new drugs, David has flourished—now a freshman in high school he is on the honor roll. His "temper tantrums" have been reduced to perhaps once per week. The neurologist would like to keep David on these medications through high school, at which time he believes that David will have developed the appropriate coping skills.

Our experiences with the medical establishment have underscored my belief that just because individuals have received their license to practice, does not mean that they are qualified to do everything.

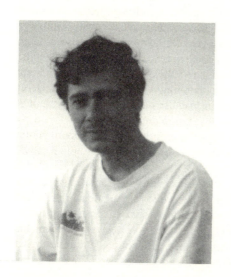

AN INTERVIEW WITH PETER TEICHMAN

I am a 33–year–old Family Practice Physician and have been licensed for two to five years. In various parts of the country where I have lived, I have treated Navaho Indians, Native Hawaiians, Tlingit Indians, Aluptick Alaskans and Mexican-Americans. I am most interested in rural health care issues and I enjoy delivering babies and caring for young families. At the time I received my medical degree, I also received a master's degree in public health administration, which included an externship at the Public Health Service in Washington, D.C. My master's thesis examined how organizational groups (like physicians, nurses and nutritionists) have advocated for the inclusion of different criteria to evaluate grant proposals in order to compete for federal funds and ultimately provide federal services to people.

To be successful wellness providers, physicians must create an atmosphere in which wisdom shows itself. This concept is expressed through the Eskimo word *Isumataq*. Doctors should allow their wisdom to show itself through communication with patients.

I have found that the best listener may learn the most. Listening enables doctors to learn a patient's baseline knowledge, beliefs, hopes, and fears. Doctors can then blend what they have learned with their own knowledge and beliefs. Doctors must discuss with patients the various options available to them in light of the combined knowledge and belief systems of both the doctor and patient. Because patients should ultimately choose which treatment to pursue, doctors should ultimately support those choices.

By working outside of my Anglo home culture I have learned how to more effectively communicate with patients from different cultural groups. Because there are no ground rules that are agreed upon, I have learned that I must be patient during any "warming up" period with ethnic persons. Doctors often expect Anglo patients to ask advice and, once it is given, to follow it. Some ethnic clients, like the Aluptik, obtain physicians' opinions and then weigh them against the opinions received from others, including their families. Whenever possible, I may acknowledge that the advice the family has given the patient is also parallel and consistent with the advice that I would give.

In situations where I believe patients are getting faulty advice, I ask them the reasons underlying this advice. If I think the reasons are faulty, I explain why I believe they are faulty.

Ethnic clients often come to Anglo physicians with hesitancy. Historically, such groups have resented the exploitation by the white race. Patients may come to physicians to see what kind of persons they are because they may anticipate being "used" or practiced upon. As a result of this situation, I have grown to be a better listener, particularly as I have realized that patients are not there to be given "marching orders" or to obtain prescriptions that must be followed to the letter. I also suspect that the native patients I have treated may be more likely to advocate for full services because they believe that non-natives do not value their lives as much as they do.

Our technological approach to health care has allowed the person to get lost in the patient. I believe that health is much more than the absence of disease. Maintaining health involves finding a way to balance one's life motivations with the physical processes that may go awry.

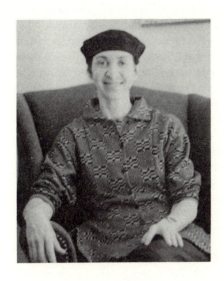

AN INTERVIEW WITH KARIN SCHNEIDER

This represents the author's interview with Ms. Schneider who lives in the rural northeast. Three weeks ago Karin's father died of liver cancer and five months ago her father-in-law also died. In both instances, she has come to respect the work of hospice staff and nurses in making the end-of-life more dignified and by offering supportive services to families. These experiences have given her the ability to compare and contrast services and care that were offered in the hospital and later through hospice.

When Ms. Schneider's father entered hospice, she was struck by how respectfully the staff treated him—they called him Mr. Schneider or by his first name. In the hospital, while her father waited for placement in a hospice, he was largely unresponsive because he slept most of the time. The nurse called him "sweetie" and treated him as if he were a child. Ms. Schneider thought that the hospital staff did not seem to be formally trained in the care of the dying, although she was pleased to see some hospitals in her area with palliative care units.

When her father was a patient in the hospice, staff would talk to him even though he was unresponsive. Although her father appeared to be unconscious one of the members of the hospice staff asked him if there was anything she could do for him. Even though he didn't respond, she then asked whether there was anything she could do for his wife. He opened his eyes and said: "That would be a good idea."

Hospice staff made a marked and conscious effort to keep the family involved in Mr. Schneider's care. Since the family was spending so much time with him, the staff would ask them whether they thought Mr. Schneider was comfortable, unlike hospital staff who never solicited the family's opinions.

After experiencing these recent deaths Karin notes a distinction between quantity versus quality of life. Life-prolonging measures the medical profession often uses in end-of-life care focus on the quantity of a patient's life. But a family's decision to place their loved one in a hospice, in which the patient will not receive life-prolonging treatment, causes the patient, family, and hospice staff to focus on the quality of the patient's remaining days. For example, the doctor of Ms. Schneider's father-in-law, who was also his friend, wanted him to live and ordered life-prolonging treatment: but the tube that went down her father-in-law's throat was very distressing to him and was certainly pointless because he knew he was dying. Her father-in-law eventually pulled out this tube. A Visiting Nurse also told the family that the intravenous fluids that were being prescribed for Karin's father-in-law were too much to handle for his system, which was shutting down, and were causing him great discomfort. After Karin's father-in-law removed the tube from his throat, he became comfortable and the next few days (only three days before his death) he was able to visit with family for many hours.

NOTES

1. This is the author's own impression on reading his medical chart even though his doctor includes psychosocial data, such as the fact that he is writing books, in his progress notes. A medical student or resident reading this chart, without an extensive conversation with the author's treating physician, probably would have no indication of what he is really like as a person.

2. Interestingly, the author suggests that this will return some pleasure to the practice of medicine.

3. These words are attributed to Confucius and are referenced in Thoreau's *Walden.*

4. The following case study illustrates the devastating effect of destroying a patient's belief in a particular therapy:

A gentleman with advanced lymph cancer had heard of Krebiozen. Although the man's doctors estimated that he had only two weeks to live, the man insisted upon being admitted into a clinical trial of the drug. Within ten days of receiving the drug, the patient's tumors had shrunk remarkably. However, two months later after the patient had heard reports containing "discouraging facts" about the drug, he made a visit to the hospital and his tumors were again enlarged. The doctor told the patient that the first batches of the drug had deteriorated in storage and that the patient would be administered a more potent shipment. At this time, the doctor injected the patient with plain water. The tumor subsequently shrank and the patient had a total remission of his symptoms. He remained healthy until he heard a news report about Krebiozen as a worthless treatment. The patient died two days later. (Klopfer, 1957)

SUGGESTED READINGS

Cousins, Norman. *Head First: The Biology of Hope.* New York: E. P. Dutton, 1989.
———. *The Healing Heart: Antidotes to Panic and Helplessness.* New York: W. W. Norton, 1983.
Hunter, Kathryn Montgomery. *Doctors' Stories: The Narrative Structure of Medical Knowledge.* Princeton, NJ: Princeton University Press, 1991.
Siegel, Bernie S. *How to Live Between Office Visits: A Guide to Life, Love, and Health.* New York: HarperCollins, 1993.
———. *Love, Medicine, and Miracles: Lessons Learned about Self-Healing from a Surgeon's Experience with Exceptional Patients.* New York: Harper & Row, 1986.

REFERENCES

Blanchard, Christina G., Mark S. Labrecque, John C. Ruckdeschel, et al. "Information and Decision Making Preferences of Hospitalized Adult Cancer Patients." 27 *Social Science and Medicine* 1139–45 (1988).
Brody, Howard. "Commentary: Hope." 246 *Journal of the American Medical Association* 1411–12 (Sept. 25, 1961).
Brown, S., A. Nelson, S. Bronkesh, et al. *Patient Satisfaction Pays: Quality Service for Practice Success.* Gaithersburg, MD: Aspen, 1993.
Broyard, Anatole. *Intoxicated by My Illness: And Other Writings on Life and Death.* New

York: Fawcett Columbine, 1993.

Callen, Michael. *Surviving AIDS*. New York: HarperCollins, 1990.

Carrese, Joseph A., and Lorna A. Rhodes. "Western Bioethics on the Navajo Reservation: Benefit or Harm?" 274 *Journal of the American Medical Association* 826–29 (Sept. 13, 1995).

Cassell, Eric. *Talking with Patients*. Vol. 1. *The Theory of Doctor-Patient Communication*. Cambridge, MA: MIT Press, 1985.

Cohan, Gary R. "Viewpoint: Two Hats." *The Advocate*, May 14, 1996, p. 47.

Cousins, Norman. *Head First: The Biology of Hope*. New York: E. P. Dutton, 1989.

———. *The Healing Heart: Antidotes to Panic and Helplessness*. New York: W. W. Norton, 1983.

Dossey, Larry. *Healing Words: The Power of Prayer and the Practice of Medicine*. San Francisco: HarperSan Francisco, 1993.

Egbert, Lawrence D., George E. Battit, Claude E. Welch, et al. "Reduction of Postoperative Pain by Encouragement and Instruction of Patients." 270 *New England Journal of Medicine* 825–27 (April 16, 1964).

Fallowfield, Leslie. "Giving Sad and Bad News." 341 *Lancet* 476–78 (1993).

Frankel, R., and H. Beckman. "Evaluating the Patient's Primary Problem(s)." In *Communicating with Medical Patients*. M. Stewart and D. Roter, eds. Newbury Park, CA: Sage, 1989, pp. 86–98.

Frankl, Viktor E. *The Doctor and the Soul: An Introduction to Logotherapy*. New York: Alfred A. Knopf, 1957.

Gallagher, Winifred. "Go with the Flow." *N.Y. Times*, Nov. 30, 1997, Sec. 7, p. 17.

Gerteis, Margaret, S. Edgman-Levitan, Jennifer Daley, et al., eds. *Through the Patient's Eyes: Understanding and Promoting Patient-Centered Care*. San Francisco: Jossey-Bass, 1993.

Hall, Judith A., and Michael C. Dornan. "What Patients Like about Their Medical Care and How Often They Are Asked: A Meta-Analysis of the Satisfaction Literature." 27 *Social Science and Medicine* 935–39 (1988).

Hall, Judith A., Arnold M. Epstein, Mary Lou DeCiantis, et al. "Physicians' Liking for Their Patients: More Evidence for the Role of Affect in Medical Care." 12 *Health Psychology* 140–46 (March 1993).

Hall, Judith A., and Debra L. Roter. "Physicians' Knowledge and Self-Reported Compliance Promotion as Predictors of Performance with Simulated Lung Disease Patients." 11 *Evaluation and the Health Professions* 306–17 (1988).

Harwood, Alan. "Mainland Puerto Ricans." In *Ethnicity and Medical Care*. A. Harwood, ed. Cambridge, MA: Harvard University Press, 1981, pp. 397–481.

Haug, Marie R., and Bebe Lavin. *Consumerism in Medicine: Challenging Physician Authority*. Beverly Hills, CA: Sage, 1983.

Hawkins, Anne Hunsaker. *Reconstructing Illness: Studies in Pathography*. West Lafayette, IN: Purdue University Press, 1993.

Hirshberg, Caryle, and Marc Ian Barasch. *Remarkable Recovery: What Extraordinary Healings Tell Us about Getting Well and Staying Well*. New York: Riverhead Books, 1995.

Hoover v. Agency for Health Care Administration, 676 So. 2d 1380, 1382 (Fla. App. 1996).

Hunter, Kathryn Montgomery. *Doctors' Stories: The Narrative Structure of Medical Knowledge*. Princeton, NJ: Princeton University Press, 1991.

Jackson, Stanley W. "The Listening Healer in the History of Psychological Healing." 149 *American Journal of Psychiatry* 1623–32 (Dec. 1992).

Jamison, Kay Redfield. *An Unquiet Mind: A Memoir of Moods and Madness*. New York:

Alfred A. Knopf, 1995.

Janiger, Oscar, and Philip Goldberg. *A Different Kind of Healing: Doctors Speak Candidly about Their Successes with Alternative Medicine.* New York: G.P. Putnam's Sons, 1993.

Kaplan, George A., and Terry Camacho. "Perceived Health and Mortality: A Nine-Year Follow-up of the Human Population Laboratory Cohort." 117 *American Journal of Epidemiology* 292–304 (1983).

Klopfer, Bruno. "Psychological Variables in Human Cancer." 21 *Journal of Projective Techniques* 331–40 (1957).

Miller, Julie. "Can One Die Not in Pain, Not in Fear?" *N.Y. Times,* Jan. 4, 1998, Sec. 14CN (Connecticut Weekly Desk), p. 1.

Mills, Mina, Huw T.O. Davies, and William A. Macrae. "Care of Dying Patients in Hospital." 309 *British Medical Journal* 583–86 (1994).

Nelson, C., and T. McLemone. *The National Ambulatory Medical Care Survey: U.S. 1975–81, and 1985 Trends.* National Center for Health Statistics. Washington, DC: U.S. Government Printing Office, 1988 (DHHS Pub. No. [PHS] 88–1954).

Olin, Harry S. "A Proposed Model to Teach Medical Students the Care of the Dying Patient." 47 *Journal of Medical Education* 564–67 (July 1972).

Oxler, Karen F. "Achieving Patient Satisfaction: Resolving Patient Complaints." 11 *Holistic Nursing Practice* 27–34 (1997).

Pelletier, Kenneth R. *Mind as Healer, Mind as Slayer: A Holistic Approach to Preventing Stress Disorders.* New York: Delta Books, 1977.

Quill, Timothy E. "Partnerships in Patient Care: A Contractual Approach." 98 *Annals of Internal Medicine* 228–34 (1983).

Rabkin, Judith G., Robert H. Remien, Lewis S. Katoff, et al. "Resilience in Adversity among Long-Term Survivors of AIDS." 44 *Hospital and Community Psychiatry* 162–67 (1993).

Redelmeier, Donald A., Jean-Pierre Molin, and Robert J. Tibshirani. "A Randomized Trial of Compassionate Care for the Homeless." 345 *Lancet* 1131–34 (May 6, 1995).

Rich, Ben A. "A Legacy of Silence: Bioethics and the Culture of Pain." 18 *Journal of Medicine and Humanities* 233 (1997).

Roter, Debra L., and Judith A. Hall. *Doctors Talking with Patients/Patients Talking with Doctors: Improving Communication in Medical Visits.* Westport, CT: Auburn House, 1993.

Rutchick, Renie. "When Pain and Policy Collide." *N.Y. Times,* Sec. A., p. 24 (letter to the editor).

Sacks, Oliver. *A Leg to Stand On.* New York: Summit Books, 1984.

Sayre, Robert F., ed. *Henry David Thoreau: A Week on the Concord and Merrimack Rivers.* New York: Library of America, 1985.

Schiff, Gordon D., Andrew B. Bindman, Troyen A. Brennan, et al. "A Better-Quality Alternative—Single Payer National Health System Reform." 272 *Journal of the American Medical Association* 803–8 (Sept. 14, 1994).

Shapiro, Robyn S. "Health Care Providers' Liability Exposure for Inappropriate Pain Management." 24 *Journal of Legal Medicine and Ethics* 360 (1996).

Sharp, David. "Difficult Patients." 12 *Hippocrates* 50–56 (1998).

Siegel, Bernie S. *How to Live Between Office Visits: A Guide to Life, Love, and Health.* New York: HarperCollins, 1993.

———. *Love, Medicine, and Miracles: Lessons Learned about Self-Healing from a Surgeon's Experience with Exceptional Patients.* New York: Harper & Row, 1986.

———. *Peace, Love, and Healing: Bodymind Communication and the Path to Self-*

Healing: An Exploration. New York: Harper & Row, 1989.

Starr, Paul. *The Social Transformation of American Medicine.* New York: Basic Books, 1982.

Stewart, M.A., and C. Buck. "Physicians' Knowledge of and Response to Patients' Problems." 15 *Medical Care* 578–85 (1977).

Stewart, Moira, Judith Belle Brown, W. Wayne Weston, et al. *Patient-Centered Medicine: Transforming the Clinical Method.* Thousand Oaks, CA: Sage Publications, 1995.

Stolberg, Sheryl Gay. "Amid New Calls for Pain Relief, New Calls for Caution." *N.Y. Times,* Oct. 13, 1998a, Sec. F, p. 7.

———. "As Life Ebbs, So Does Time to Elect Comforts of Hospice." *N.Y. Times,* March 4, 1998b, Sec. A, p. 1.

———. "Study Finds Pain of Oldest Is Ignored In Nursing Homes." *N.Y. Times,* June 17, 1998c, Sec. A, p. 1.

Thomas, K.B. "General Practice Considerations: Is There Any Point in Being Positive?" 294 *British Medical Journal* 1200–1202 (1987).

Tuckett, David, Coral Olson Boulton, and Anthony Williams. *Meetings Between Experts: An Approach to Sharing Ideas in Medical Consultations.* New York: Tavistock, 1985.

Wade, Nicholas. "The Spin Doctors." *N.Y. Times Magazine,* Jan. 7, 1996, p. 16.

Warren, Elizabeth. "Aftermath: One Woman's Story of a Little-Known Risk in Breast Cancer Surgery." *Chicago Tribune Magazine,* June 23, 1996, Sec. 10, pp. 13 et. seq.

Watson, J. *Nursing: Human Science and Human Care: A Theory of Nursing,* 2nd ed. New York: National League for Nursing, 1988.

Weinberg, Richard B. "Shelter from the Storm." *The New Physician* 13–14 (Dec. 1988).

Wolf, Stewart. "The Pharmacology of Placebos." 11 *Pharmacological Reviews* 689–704 (1959).

Zinsser, Hans. *As I Remember Him: The Biography of R.S.* Boston: Little, Brown, 1940.

7

Legal Issues in the Health Care Setting

INTRODUCTION

Many legal issues arise in the health care setting, such as the nature of the disclosure that doctors need to make about the procedures and treatments patients will undergo; the right of patients to execute documents called *advance directives*, typically including "living wills" or "powers of attorney"; and issues related to the right to die, including whether patients have any right to physician-assisted suicide.

The requirement that doctors disclose to patients information about the procedures and treatments they will undergo stems from the legal doctrine of *informed consent*, which ensures that patients have as much information as possible so that their decisions will reflect their wishes regarding their health-related care. The doctrine also ensures that patients are not subjected to procedures that they do not want to undergo and, therefore, actually protects patients from unwarranted intrusions upon their bodies. Such an intrusion is legally defined as a *battery*.

The right of patients to execute advance directives is expressly recognized by most states. In supporting patients' rights to execute such documents, states protect patients' autonomy and allow them to make decisions involving end-of-life issues, particularly with regard to the use of artificial means of support and the provision of food and water to sustain (or prolong) life.

Issues related to the right to die have been litigated in the court system for many years, particularly since the 1970s. Although many of these cases have been decided by state courts, many others have been reviewed by the Supreme Court of the United States.

THE LEGAL IMPLICATIONS OF COMMUNICATION
BETWEEN DOCTORS AND PATIENTS

What doctors have told patients about their health status has changed dramatically over time, at least in the United States, and varies widely from culture to culture. In 1961, a landmark study in the United States noted that 90 percent of surgeons would not routinely discuss a patient's cancer diagnosis (Oken, 1961). Yet by 1979, more than 90 percent of physicians in the United States said they would tell their patients if they had cancer (Novack, Plumer, Smith, et al., 1979).

Although physicians in the United States often disclose much information to patients about their health status, such levels of disclosure do not necessarily occur in other industrialized cultures (Mitchell, 1998). A 1993 study showed that 63 percent of European gastroenterologists did not routinely disclose a cancer diagnosis to patients if the patient did not ask for the results (Thomsen, Wulff, Martin, et al., 1993). Similarly, a survey of British medical practitioners and hospital consultants in the early 1980s found that 75 and 56 percent, respectively, did not routinely tell their patients of their diagnoses (Wilkes, 1984). In Japan, patients have traditionally not been informed of a diagnosis of cancer (Sasako, 1996) or even HIV infection (Aoki, Ngin, Mo, et al., 1989); a 1995 survey of the Ministry of Health and Welfare revealed that only 20 percent of patients who had recently died of cancer were told their diagnosis (Sasako, 1996). But as the highlight box "Informed Consent in Japan" on the following page indicates, this situation is changing.

Legal Standards for the Disclosure of Information about Procedures

There are two different standards courts use to examine the sufficiency of the disclosures doctors make to patients: the professional community and the informed consent standards. Under the *professional community standard*, a court considers whether the nature of a disclosure physicians make to patients is what reasonable medical practitioners would disclose (Annas, 1989, p. 241). Under the *informed consent standard*, courts look to whether a reasonable patient would consider the nature of what is to be disclosed "material" (ibid., p. 86). If the facts to be disclosed are material, the law would require disclosure. The doctrine of informed consent has been the hallmark for judging the adequacy of physician disclosures to patients regarding the risks or benefits of various tests, procedures, and medications. Courts have an increased tendency to apply the informed consent standard.

Courts have not imposed legal liability upon physicians for disclosing too much information to a patient (Annas, 1989), but physicians have been held liable for disclosing too little information. Consider some situations in which doctors would disclose too little information to patients. Since most physicians believe that there is one preferred treatment option and that patients' health would be jeopardized if an alternative were chosen (Lidz, Meisel, Osterweis, et al., 1983), physicians may not fully describe procedures or treatments of which they do not approve. Furthermore, it is possible that physicians may not tell patients about alternate procedures or surgeries that they do not perform—hence, they may fail to make an appropriate referral.

INFORMED CONSENT IN JAPAN

In Japan there is no legal requirement that doctors inform patients of the nature of their illnesses. Japan's Supreme Court has ruled that doctors are not required to tell patients if they are suffering from cancer (Sterngold, 1992). This holding defers to the traditional role of doctors—to tell the patient's family that the patient has cancer and let the family decide on whether it is appropriate to tell the patient (Ohnuki-Tierney, 1984, p. 216). Historically, the doctor/patient relationship in Japan has been considered quite paternalistic. Some scholars argue that paternalism was fostered by the fact that "the Japanese expect others without verbal communication to consider what they need and unconsciously require [them] to act in their best interest" (Atsushi, Kishino, Fukui, et al., 1998).

Recent studies suggest, however, that the doctor/patient relationship in Japan is changing—and much of this change is motivated by Japanese patients who are dissatisfied with their doctors (ibid.). In the study mentioned, 56 percent of the 286 respondents had changed their previous physicians because they were not satisfied with the physician's explanations regarding diagnostic procedures or treatments. Furthermore:

- Of respondents who complained about their physicians' explanations 66 percent claimed they were too difficult to understand (n = 298).
- Of the respondents, 39 percent had difficulty understanding the physicians' explanation regarding prognosis.
- In addition, 34 percent could not understand the possible adverse effects of treatment.

It is quite possible that Japanese patients who are unsatisfied with their physicians will change doctors to avoid confrontation (see Nilchaikovit, Hill, & Holland, 1993) rather than stay with and attempt to persuade their doctor.

Patients taking experimental drugs in Japan are not always told that they are participating in trials (Sterngold, 1992), and doctors frequently remove the labels from prescription drugs, so, in fact, patients may have no idea of the drugs they are taking (ibid.). In the United States, such practices would obviously raise significant issues related to informed consent.

The law is unsettled as to whether doctors must disclose a prognosis to patients, although this question becomes more complicated when one considers the issue of whether patients would opt for different therapies had their prognoses been disclosed. Some studies indicate that patients prefer to be told their prognosis (Kindelan & Kent, 1987).

At least one suit considered whether a doctor is obliged to disclose a patient's prognosis so that the patient can get his or her affairs "in order." In *Arato v. Avedon* (1993), the Supreme Court of California confronted the issue of whether a patient's treating doctors should be liable for not disclosing a cancer patient's statistical life expectancy (SLE). Although the court said that doctors must disclose information regarding the significant risks associated with treatments, revealing additional information like SLE could not be mandated as a matter of law but must depend upon the standard practice in the medical community. Representatives for the deceased patient, who had pancreatic cancer, had argued that the patient might not have consented to undergo chemotherapy and radiation had he understood the shortcomings of such treatments—that only 5 to 10 percent of patients with such cancer live for five years. But doctors testified during trial that the patient and his wife did not ask for information regarding SLE in over 70 visits during the year and presumably were told that most victims of pancreatic cancer died of the disease. Both the court and the testimony of the deceased patient's treating physicians indicated that statistical morbidity rates of various population groups could not reliably predict the fate of individual patients. The court would not require doctors to disclose "every contingency that might affect the patient's nonmedical 'rights and interests'" and, therefore, rejected the family's contention that the deceased needed to know his SLE to get his affairs in order.

Liability for Not Disclosing the Risk for Genetic Defects

Physicians may face liability for not disclosing the likelihood that parents will have children with certain genetic disorders. This liability varies in the different states, depending on whether the states recognize either wrongful birth or wrongful life suits. *Wrongful birth suits*, recognized in most states, are those in which parents allege that they would not have allowed their children to be born had they known in advance the children's likelihood of being born with a genetic defect. *Wrongful life suits*, recognized in a few states (e.g., California,[1] New Jersey,[2] and Washington[3]), are those in which children allege that they would not have wanted to be born to face the tremendous physical and emotional suffering they now face.

PATIENTS' RIGHTS TO SELF-DETERMINATION

Advance Directives: Powers of Attorney and Living Wills

When ill persons are not legally competent to make their own health-related decisions, any advance directive (living will or power of attorney for health care) that they executed prior to their incompetence is to be honored and respected by health care professionals (for further information, see the highlight box "Basic Information Often Contained in Powers of Attorney for Health Care"). There is an important distinction between medical competence and legal competence. Even though patients are not medically competent to make decisions, they may be legally competent to make them. For purposes of the law, the mental capacity to execute such a document (called *testamentary capacity*) means that the principal has "sufficient mind and memory to intelligently understand the nature of the business in which he is engaged, [can] comprehend generally the nature and extent of the property which constitutes his estate, and which he intends to dispose of, and to recollect the objects of his bounty" (*Black's Law Dictionary*, 1979, p. 1322). Although persons may be confused, suffering from dementia, or receiving life support, this does not mean that they lack the mental capacity needed to execute a valid power of attorney for health care or a living will (see Annas, 1989, p. 201) (being "mentally retarded or committed to a mental hospital does not automatically render the person incompetent").

Although it is advisable that all persons execute advance directives while they are competent, certain groups of persons should be particularly aware of their need to do so. These groups include persons estranged from their families, such as some gays and lesbians, who might want a close friend, neighbor, or lover to act on their behalf if they become incompetent.[4] Even near the time of death, however, families may want to control one's "final" affairs and may strongly resent that one's friend, neighbor, or lover has the power to make life and death decisions.

The validity of powers of attorney can be contested in court proceedings for some of the following reasons:

- The principal did not have the required mental capacity to execute the document.
- The agent procured his or her agency via fraud.
- The agent did not act in the principal's best interest.

A principal must have the appropriate mental capacity to execute a power of attorney at the time the document is executed. Agents who are not acting in the principal's best interest can be removed from their role and the court will instead appoint a guardian to make the principal's health-related decisions. The fact that family members do not like or trust nominated agents does not automatically mean that they are not acting in the principal's best interest. But

BASIC INFORMATION OFTEN CONTAINED IN POWERS OF ATTORNEY FOR HEALTH CARE

Powers of attorney for health care frequently contain information with regard to the following:

- Any restriction in the type of medical or other procedures that may be performed in the event of the disability of the principal—the person executing the document.
- Information as to the proper disposition of the body at death (e.g., whether the principal prefers to be cremated or consent to an autopsy).
- Information as to when the power will become effective (consider having the document become effective when a specific doctor or doctors certify that the principal is no longer physically/mentally able to make his or her health-related decisions).
- Information when the power will terminate.
- The name of the person who will be invested with decision-making authority (the agent) when the principal is no longer competent.
- The names of persons who will be successor agents in the event the named agent is not able to or is unwilling to act.

Principals must remember that powers of attorney for health care are merely "pieces of paper" that may not be recognized by health care professionals (HCPs) even though they are legally binding documents. To ensure that an advance directive is followed, principals must appoint an assertive agent—known to the principal and familiar with the types of health-related decisions he or she is likely to prefer.

Agents may need to be assertive because they may need to challenge the authority of HCPs who may not want to give effect to a health care power. This agent may need to remind HCPs of their possible legal liability for failure to carry out the wishes expressed in a power of attorney.

It is generally not recommended that powers of attorney state a date on which they terminate, because on that date, the principal may be incompetent and unable to execute a new document.

of course such dislike or distrust may not necessarily prevent such family members from bringing a lawsuit. In one case, *In Re Guardianship of Sharon Kowalski* (1991), one member of a lesbian couple sued to be the guardian/caretaker of her lover of at least three years before the lover was critically injured in a car accident. The father of the injured lover sought to become guardian; in so doing, he denied his daughter's lesbianism and the fact that her lover had a legitimate interest in her welfare. Thompson, the partner, faced a court battle of nine and a half years in order to be legally entitled to make decisions about her lover's health care. She also had to sue just to visit her incapacitated lover because the law did not recognize her as a "family" member.

A living will is a second type of advance directive, which instructs physicians not to use death-delaying procedures when one is diagnosed as having a condition that makes death imminent. The living will is merely an *instruction* to physicians—they are not mandated to honor the requests of a patient's living will (Annas, 1989, p. 210). Although there is no absolute certainty as to what procedures are death-delaying, states may allow individuals to refuse "extraordinary" or "artificial" treatments. Most states require, however, that only the "terminally ill" are covered by living will statutes (ibid., p. 209).

One of the most significant problems related to advance directives may be their vague language. As two astute commentators have queried "What does 'heroic' or 'extraordinary' mean for a particular patient in a particular set of circumstances?" (Schoene-Seifert & Childress, 1986).

Despite the Patient Self-Determination Act of 1990, a federal law that requires hospitals to inform patients about their rights to establish advance directives, physicians are reluctant to raise the issue but are willing to discuss it if the patient asks (Morrison, Morrison, & Glickman, 1994).

In catastrophic situations, it is "disturbing" that physicians report "little use" of advance directives to guide their treatment decisions (ibid.). Unfortunately, HCPs routinely ignore legally valid advance directives (Danis, Southerland, Garrett, et al., 1991) and either substitute their ideas about what they believe should be done under the circumstances or defer to the wishes of family members who may not have the same legal authority as an agent under a power of attorney. Physicians impose their wishes regarding end-of-life decisions more than 60 percent of the time, even when those wishes are expressly contrary to the written advance directives of patients (ibid.). In order to ensure that a health care power will be enforced, principals must choose an assertive agent who can run "interference" with hospital staff or family members so that their wishes are honored.

Cardiopulmonary Resuscitation and "Do Not Resuscitate" Orders

Many advance directives are silent about the principal's preferences regarding cardiopulmonary resuscitation (CPR), even though cardiac arrest occurs during the dying process of each person. Apparently, it is uncommon for physicians to solicit a patient's feedback regarding any preference for CPR.

In a study of 154 patients resuscitated at Boston's Beth Israel Hospital in 1981, physicians had an opinion about the patient's wishes in 68 percent of the cases, but only 30 patients (19 percent) had discussed resuscitation with a physician before their cardiac arrest (Bedell & Delbanco, 1984).[5] This information may raise more questions than it answers, such as

- Is it reasonable to assume that patients do not want to be resuscitated if their powers of attorney for health care stipulated that they do not want any "death-delaying" procedures used?
- Even if patients have such advance directives, shouldn't doctors specifically discuss CPR with them?

Although patients may legally refuse CPR, as they can any other medical intervention, the medical practice "seems to be that no one can die in a hospital without CPR" (Annas, 1989, p. 216). Because doctors have a legal privilege to treat patients in "emergencies" without their consent (ibid.), during an "emergency" they would not have to get consent to perform CPR.

THE RIGHT TO DIE

Some Definitions

Before discussing the issue of the right to die, essentially euthanasia, we must distinguish between active and passive euthanasia, terms that were commonly used in the 1950s and 1960s (Reich, 1995, p. 565). *Active euthanasia*, which includes physician-assisted suicide, is a "deliberate intervention to end a patient's life—by administering a lethal injection" (ibid.). *Passive euthanasia* was understood as forgoing "life sustaining treatment either by stopping it or not starting it" (ibid.). Passive euthanasia has apparently occurred in medicine for a long time, although only recently have doctors begun to talk openly about it.

History of the Right to Die Movement

The right to die movement started in the United States in the mid-1970s, when courts reviewed cases brought on behalf of terminally ill persons—often in comas and on respirators—seeking their right to die.[6] At issue in these cases was who was responsible for making medical decisions for incompetent persons who had neither expressed their wishes regarding death-delaying procedures nor executed advance directives. Often HCPs disagreed with family members as to whether heroic measures should be continued, at least when the incompetent person had poor "quality of life." Presumably, 80 percent of physicians favor withdrawing life-support systems "from hopelessly ill or irreversibly comatose patients if they or their families request it" (Annas, 1989, p. 223).

Although these types of cases still present thorny issues, some states have passed statutes to assist courts to determine who shall make health-related decisions for incompetent patients in the absence of a health care power of attorney. In Illinois, for example, the Health Care Surrogate Act provides that "surrogate decision makers" can make decisions, without judicial involvement, on behalf of patients who lack the "decisional capacity to terminate life sustaining treatment."[7] The act also stipulates that these decision makers shall make decisions for adult patients that conform "to what the patient would have done or intended under the circumstances," taking into account the patient's personal, philosophical, religious, moral, and ethical beliefs. The surrogate is also charged with determining how a patient would have weighed the burdens and benefits of initiating or continuing life–sustaining treatment against the benefits and burdens of that treatment.

Many of these early, and subsequent, right to die decisions seemed to indicate that incompetent patients had a right to autonomy, a personal right to determine the dignity of their death. As a result, experts in the field thought that the Supreme Court of the United States would protect this "autonomy interest" as it did previous interests, such as the right to decide to have an abortion (*Roe v. Wade*, 1973) or "to bear or beget a child" (*Eisenstadt v. Baird*, 1972).

In the United States, there is no constitutionally recognized right to die per se. In *Cruzan v. Director, Missouri Department of Health* (1990), the Court found that there was a constitutionally protected "liberty" interest in allowing competent persons the right to refuse lifesaving hydration and nutrition. The Court's reasoning was based on the common law notion that forced medication is a battery (the legal term for an unpermitted bodily touching or intrusion); therefore, patients had a long-recognized right to refuse unwanted treatment.

Physician-Assisted Suicide: Views from the Supreme Court and the Medical Profession

In *Washington v. Glucksberg* (1997), however, the Court found that there was no constitutionally protected right to have a physician assist a patient to commit suicide.

Washington v. Glucksberg: Chief Justice Rehnquist delivered the opinion of the Court
The question presented in this case is whether [the state of] Washington's prohibition against "caus[ing]" or "aid[ing]" a suicide offends the Fourteenth Amendment to the United States Constitution. We hold that it does not.
We begin, as we do in all due-process cases, by examining our Nation's history, legal traditions, and practices. In almost every State—indeed, in almost every western democracy—it is a crime to assist a suicide. The States' assisted-suicide bans . . . are longstanding expressions of the States' commitment to the protection and preservation of all human life. Moreover, the majority of States in this country have laws imposing criminal penalties on one who assists another to commit suicide. . . . [T]he prohibitions against assisting suicide never contained exceptions for those who were near death. Rather, "[t]he life of those to whom life ha[d] become a burden—of those who [were] hopelessly diseased or fatally wounded—nay, even the lives of criminals condemned to death, [were] under the protection of law, equally as the lives of those who [were] in the full tide of life's enjoyment, and anxious to continue to live."
California voters rejected an assisted-suicide initiative similar to Washington's in 1993. On the other hand, in 1994, voters in Oregon enacted, also through ballot initiative, that State's "Death With Dignity Act," which legalized physician-assisted suicide for

competent, terminally ill adults. Since the Oregon vote, many proposals to legalize assisted-suicide have been and continue to be introduced in the States' legislatures, but none have been enacted. . . . Also, on April 30, 1997, President Clinton signed the Federal Assisted Suicide Funding Restriction Act of 1997, which prohibits the use of federal funds in support of physician-assisted suicide.

The Due Process Clause guarantees more than fair process, and the "liberty" it protects includes more than the absence of physical restraint. In a long line of cases, we have held that, in addition to the specific freedoms protected by the Bill of Rights, the "liberty" specially protected by the Due Process Clause includes the rights to marry, to have children, to direct the education and upbringing of one's children, to marital privacy, to use contraception, to bodily integrity, and to abortion. We have also assumed, and strongly suggested, that the Due Process Clause protects the traditional right to refuse unwanted life-saving medical treatment. (*Cruzan*)

Turning to the claim at issue here, the Court of Appeals stated that "[p]roperly analyzed, the first issue to be resolved is whether there is a liberty interest in determining the time and manner of one's death," or, in other words, "[i]s there a right to die?" Similarly, respondents assert a "liberty to choose how to die" and a right to "control of one's final days," and describe the asserted liberty as "the right to choose a humane, dignified death," and "the liberty to shape death." . . . [A]lthough *Cruzan* is often described as a "right to die" case, we were, in fact, more precise: we assumed that the Constitution granted competent persons a "constitutionally protected right to refuse lifesaving hydration and nutrition." The Washington statute at issue in this case prohibits "aid[ing] another person to attempt suicide," and, thus, the question before us is whether the "liberty" specially protected by the Due Process Clause includes a right to commit suicide which itself includes a right to assistance in doing so.

We now inquire whether this asserted right has any place in our Nation's traditions. [The Court notes an almost "universal tradition" which has rejected the asserted right.]

Respondents contend, however, that the liberty interest they assert is consistent with this Court's substantive-due-process line of cases. . . . Pointing to *Casey* and *Cruzan*, respondents read our jurisprudence in this area as reflecting a general tradition of "self-sovereignty" and as teaching that the "liberty" protected by the Due Process Clause includes "basic and intimate exercises of personal autonomy." According to respondents our liberty jurisprudence . . . protects the "liberty of competent, terminally ill adults to make end-of-life decisions free of undue government interference."

The right assumed in *Cruzan*, however, was not simply deduced from abstract concepts of personal autonomy. Given the common-law rule that forced medication was a battery, and the long legal tradition protecting the decision to refuse unwanted medical treatment, our assumption was entirely consistent with this Nation's history and constitutional traditions. The decision to commit suicide with the assistance of another may be just as personal and profound as the decision to refuse unwanted medical treatment, but it has never enjoyed similar legal protection.

The Constitution also requires, however, that Washington's assisted-suicide ban be rationally related to legitimate government interests. This requirement is unquestionably met here. . . . Washington's assisted-suicide ban implicates a number of state interests.

[The Court notes that Washington has an "unqualified interest in the preservation of human life."]

Respondents admit that "[t]he State has a real interest in preserving the lives of those who can still contribute to society and enjoy life." The Court of Appeals also recognized Washington's interest in protecting life, but held that the "weight" of this interest depends on the "medical condition and the wishes of the person whose life is at stake." Washington, however, has rejected this sliding-scale approach and, through its assisted-suicide ban, insists that all persons' lives, from beginning to end, regardless of physical or mental condition, are under the full protection of the law. [T]he States "may properly make judgments about the 'quality' of life that a particular individual may enjoy."

[The Court notes research and data that many people who request physician-assisted suicide withdraw that request if their depression and pain are treated.]

The State also has an interest in protecting the integrity and ethics of the medical profession. [P]hysician-assisted suicide could, it is argued, undermine the trust that is essential to the doctor-patient relationship by blurring the time-honored line between healing and harming.

Next, the State has an interest in protecting vulnerable groups—including the poor, the elderly, and disabled persons—from abuse, neglect, and mistakes.

The State's interest here goes beyond protecting the vulnerable from coercion; it extends to protecting disabled and terminally ill people from prejudice, negative and inaccurate stereotypes, and "societal indifference." The State's assisted-suicide ban reflects and reinforces a policy that the lives of terminally ill, disabled, and elderly people must be no less valued than the lives of the young and healthy. . . .

Finally, the State may fear that permitting assisted suicide will start it down the path to voluntary and perhaps even involuntary euthanasia.

[The Court reviews research from the Netherlands that indicates that, for example, in 1990 there were 2,300 cases of voluntary euthanasia ("the deliberate termination of another's life at his request"); 400 cases of assisted suicide, and more than 1,000 cases of euthanasia without an explicit request. Furthermore, there were an additional 4,941 cases where physicians administered lethal morphine overdoses without the patients' explicit consent.]

Throughout the Nation, Americans are engaged in an earnest and profound debate about the morality, legality, and practicality of physician-assisted suicide. Our holding permits this debate to continue, as it should in a democratic society.

The *Glucksberg* Court left some questions unanswered and may have failed to give the nation's judges clear guidance in resolving future cases. Some of the justices seemed to disagree as to whether it would be legal for doctors to give patients doses of pain medication that would hasten their deaths. In her separate opinion concurring with the majority's decision, Justice O'Connor noted that palliative care is legal even when it would hasten a patient's death.[8]

Justice Stevens envisioned situations in which physician-assisted suicide would seem appropriate and entitled to constitutional protection. He suggested that in certain circumstances individuals may decide the time of their death, particularly if they were not victimized by abuse and did not suffer from depression. Justice Stevens argued that the state did not have a sufficient legitimate interest in preventing suicide of abused or depressed persons—as it did for the elderly, disabled, and other individuals who were vulnerable.

Justice Souter's concurring decision indicated that legislatures, not courts, were better equipped to deal with the question of physician-assisted suicide because legislators have "superior opportunities to obtain the facts." Nonetheless, Justice Souter noted that there are several reasons for claiming that the right to physician-assisted suicide "falls within the accepted tradition of medical care in our society" (138 L.Ed. 2d at 825). Justice Souter likened physician-assisted suicide to abortion. Even though a state has a legitimate interest in discouraging abortion, he noted the Supreme Court has recognized a woman's right to a physician's counsel and care. He reasoned that without a physician's assistance in abortion, a woman's right would "too often amount to nothing more than a right to self-mutilation." Justice Souter then observed that doctors have a role to minister to their patients. He seemed to suggest that in cases involving physician-assisted suicide doctors can fulfill this role. In such cases patients not only seek an end to their pain "but an end to their short remaining lives with a dignity that they believed would be denied them by powerful pain medication, as well as by their consciousness of dependency and helplessness as they approached death."

Certain doctors support and practice physician-assisted suicide—these doctors are more likely to treat persons with terminal illnesses, such as AIDS and cancer (Henry, 1997). As the chart below indicates, not only are doctors receiving a significant number of requests for euthanasia and physician-assisted suicide, but an appreciable percentage of them *admit* to engaging in such practices.

Country	Doctors Receiving Requests for Euthanasia & Physician-Assisted Suicide	Doctors Engaging in Such Practices
Denmark	30%	5% (Folker, Holtug, Jensen, et al., 1996)
South Australia	33%	19% (Stevens & Hassan, 1994)
United Kingdom	45%	14% (Ward & Tate, 1994)
United States	57%	14% (Emanuel, Fairclough, Daniels, et al., 1996)
Oregon	21%	7% (Lee, Nelson, Tilden et al., 1995)
Washington	16%	24% (Black, Wallace, Starks, et al., 1996)

Regardless of whether one considers physician-assisted suicide appropriate, some recent polls raise troubling questions. For example, in a survey of Oregon psychiatrists only 6 percent were very confident that in a single evaluation they could "adequately assess whether a psychiatric disorder was impairing the judgment of a patient requesting assisted suicide" (Ganzini, Fenn, Lee, et al., 1996). Depression, for example, would invalidate a patient's request for physician-assisted suicide. When many psychiatrists are unsure of whether they could adequately assess whether a patient's judgment were impaired, one wonders about the ability of other physicians to make such assessments.

There is clearly a right to physician-assisted suicide in the Netherlands (van der Maas, van Delden, Pinjnenborg, et al., 1991). The penal code in the Netherlands in the 1990s states, "Anyone who takes another's life, even upon that person's serious and explicit request, can be imprisoned for up to 12 years" (Reich, 1995, p. 561). However, the Dutch made it possible for doctors to end lives of "incurably sick and suffering patients" if they acted in accord with criteria developed in case law and established as precise guidelines in Holland's medical institutions (ibid.). These guidelines hold that patients "must be incurably sick, must be experiencing unbearable suffering and must clearly and persistently request that their lives be ended" (ibid.). In 1994, the Dutch Supreme Court ruled that in exceptional instances, physician-assisted suicide might even be justifiable for patients with unbearable mental suffering but no physical illness (Groenewoud, van der Maas, van der Wal, et al., 1997).

Critics of Holland's physician-assisted suicide law point out, however, that

- guidelines for euthanasia are not followed in more than 40 percent of euthanasia cases (van der Maas, van Delden, Pinjnenborg, et al., 1991).
- euthanasia is performed on patients who are not able either to request it or to consent to it, such as babies with birth defects and patients in persistent vegetative states (see Hendin, Rutenfrans, & Zylicz, 1997).

CHAPTER SUMMARY

Some of the many legal issues that arise in health care settings include the nature of the disclosure that doctors must make about the procedures and treatments patients will undergo, the right of patients to execute "advance directives," and issues related to the right to die, including physician-assisted suicide.

Although many states have laws that permit patients to execute advance directives, these documents can be subject to various legal challenges, may conflict with hospital "do not resuscitate" orders, and may not be recognized by hospital personnel at the end of the patient's life. Advance directives can be challenged for many of the same reasons that an individual's will can be challenged, including the fact that the person signing the directive lacked the proper mental capacity at the time it was signed. When gays and lesbians have indicated their preference that their lovers or partners be allowed to make end-of-life decisions, family members unwilling to accept the principal's homosexuality have often waged bitter court battles, usually alleging that the chosen agent did not act in the "best interests" of the principal. Furthermore, when individuals become incapacitated or incompetent, hospital personnel do not always give full effect to advance directives. For example, they often aim to "please" or indulge the wishes of the family, particularly when an agent who is not a family member has preferences opposite to those of the family.

Hospital policies regarding "do not resuscitate" orders (including cardiopulmonary resuscitation orders) can be at odds with the wishes patients have specified in their advance directives. Although advance directives give patients a heightened level of autonomy, doctors, unfortunately, do not always discuss end-of-life decisions with patients and, therefore, ignore a patient's right to autonomy. In one study in which patients were resuscitated, doctors had discussed the patient's wishes for resuscitation in only 19 percent of the cases.

In the United States there is no constitutional right to die per se, although the Supreme Court of the United States has upheld the right of competent persons to refuse lifesaving nutrition and hydration. And in *Washington v. Glucksberg*, the Court found that there was no constitutional right to physician-assisted suicide— although it upheld the right of states to pass laws permitting physician-assisted suicide. The Court noted that it would be inappropriate to sanction physician-assisted suicide because suicide is illegal in all of the states, the states have many bona fide reasons to "preserve and protect" human life, and the medical profession's role is to promote healing. However, doctors increasingly receive patients' requests for physician-assisted suicide, and many are complying with these requests. In San Francisco, for example, a survey of doctors who treat people with HIV/AIDS revealed that more than 50 percent had helped at least one patient die.

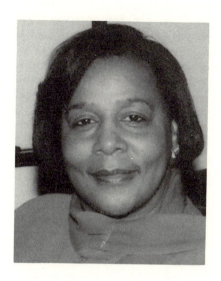

AN INTERVIEW WITH LEVORN MCCAIN-JONES

I work in a small community hospital where 90 percent of the patients are African American. Most of the doctors practicing at this hospital are foreign-born. I've worked as a nurse anesthetist for 27 years. I was also diagnosed with breast cancer for which I had a lumpectomy.

As an African American woman, I know that some black ministers encourage their church members to deny any health-related concerns. For example, I have heard some black ministers advise congregants with cancer to just "pray about it." The implication is that medical treatment is not needed. This philosophy also is the reason some elderly African Americans do not take their medication for diabetes.

More African American women die of breast cancer than Caucasian women because they seek treatment during late stages of the disease and possibly because they have reduced access to care.

As a nurse anesthetist, my job requires that I assess the risks that anesthesia may pose to patients. Prior to surgery, many patients have asked me the nature of the surgical procedure they will undergo. I often wonder whether their physicians have adequately described the nature of the procedure to them. I once talked to a woman who thought she was hospitalized for further tests but was scheduled to have a hysterectomy. It is also possible that patients may not have *heard* or understood what their doctors have told them. Consequently, doctors may have explained procedures thoroughly to patients. I often wonder whether the foreign-born doctors who practice in our hospital are able to communicate effectively with patients because sometimes it seems that it is difficult for them to communicate in English.

I believe that patients are being more assertive than they once were. For example, I've seen more patients sign themselves out of the hospital "Against Medical Advice."

Because I was diagnosed with Stage I breast cancer, I had a lumpectomy, which is much less radical than a mastectomy. I have observed, however, that all of the surgeons with whom I've worked, all perform mastectomies. I have never assisted with a lumpectomy in the 27 years I've worked at this particular hospital. I believe that if these doctors more carefully explained the different types of surgery available for the different stages of breast cancer, and encouraged patients to be more actively involved in their health care, women patients would sometimes opt for lumpectomies.

NOTES

1. *Turpin v. Sortini*, 31 Cal.3d 22, 643 P.2d 954 (1982).
2. *Procanik v. Cillo*, 97 N.J. 339, 478 A.2d 755 (1984).
3. *Harbeson v. Parke-Davis*, 98 Wash. 2d 460, 656 P.2d 483 (1983).
4. One study indicated that 47 percent of gay men wanted their partners to make decisions regarding life-sustaining treatment (Steinbrook, Lo, Moulton, et al., 1986).
5. The families of the patients were consulted in 33 percent of the cases (51 cases).
6. The two most famous cases litigated in this area are the case of Karen Ann Quinlan (see *In Re Quinlan*, 1976) and the case of Joseph Saikewicz (*Superintendent of Belchertown v. Saikewicz*, 1977).
7. There are eight categories of persons, in order of preference, listed in the Illinois statute who can qualify as surrogate decision makers: close friends of the patient are listed seventh. This has led some law review commentators to express the opinion that the Illinois legislature again rejected domestic partners' rights (Closen & Maloney, 1995).
8. With respect to palliative care, Justice Stevens noted expert opinion that as death becomes more imminent, pain and suffering become progressively more difficult to treat. See 138 L.Ed 2d at 805.

SUGGESTED READING

Annas, George. *The Rights of Patients: The Basic ACLU Guide to Patient Rights*, 2nd ed. Carbondale: Southern Illinois University Press, 1989.

REFERENCES

Annas, George. *The Rights of Patients: The Basic ACLU Guide to Patient Rights*, 2nd ed. Carbondale: Southern Illinois University Press, 1989.
Aoki, Bart, Chiang Peng Ngin, Bertha Mo, et al. "AIDS Prevention Model in Asian-American Communities." In *Primary Prevention of AIDS: Psychological Approaches*. V.M. Mays, G.W. Albee, and S.F. Schneider, eds. Newbury Park, CA: Sage, 1989, pp. 290–308.
Arato v. Avedon, 5 Cal. 4th 1172, 23 Cal. Rptr. 2d 131, 858 P.2d 598 (1993).
Atsushi, Asai, Minako Kishino, Tsuguya Fukui, et al. "Choices of Japanese Patients in the Face of Disagreement." 12 *Bioethics* 162–72 (1998).
Bedell, Susanna E., and Thomas L. Delbanco. "Choices about Cardiopulmonary Resuscitation in the Hospital: When Do Physicians Talk with Patients?" 310 *New England Journal of Medicine* 1089–93 (April 26, 1984).
Black, Anthony L., Jeffrey I. Wallace, Helene E. Starks, et al. "Physician-Assisted Suicide and Euthanasia in Washington State: Patient Requests and Physician Responses." 275 *Journal of the American Medical Association* 919–25 (March 27, 1996).
Black's Law Dictionary. 5th ed. St. Paul, MN: West Publishing, 1979.
Closen, Michael L., and Joan E. Maloney. "Health Care Surrogate Act in Illinois: Another Rejection of Domestic Partners' Rights." 19 *Southern Illinois University Law Journal* 479 (Spring 1995).
Cruzan v. Director, Missouri Department of Health, 497 U.S. 261 (1990).
Danis, Marion, Leslie I. Southerland, Joanne M. Garrett, et al. "A Prospective Study of

Advance Directives for Life-Sustaining Care." 324 *New England Journal of Medicine* 882–88 (March 28, 1991).

Eisenstadt v. Baird, 405 U.S. 438 (1972).

Emanuel, Ezekiel J., Diane L. Fairclough, Elisabeth R. Daniels, et al. "Euthanasia and Physician-Assisted Suicide: Attitudes and Experiences of Oncology Patients, Oncologists and the Public." 347 *Lancet* 1805–10 (1996).

Folker, Anna P., Nils Holtug, Annette B. Jensen, et al. "Experiences and Attitudes Towards End-of-Life Decisions Amongst Danish Physicians." 10 *Bioethics* 233–49 (1996).

Ganzini, Linda, Darien S. Fenn, Melinda A. Lee, et al. "Attitudes of Oregon Psychiatrists Toward Physician-Assisted Suicide." 153 *American Journal of Psychiatry* 1469–75 (Nov. 1996).

Groenewoud, Johanna H., Paul J. van der Maas, Gerrit van der Wal, et al. "Physician-Assisted Death in Psychiatric Practice in the Netherlands." 336 *New England Journal of Medicine* 1795–801 (June 19, 1997).

Harbeson v. Parke-Davis, 98 Wash. 2d 460, 656 P.2d 483 (1983).

Hendin, Herbert, C. Rutenfrans, and Z. Zylicz. "Physician-Assisted Suicide and Euthanasia in the Netherlands: Lessons from the Dutch." 277 *Journal of the American Medical Association* 1720–722 (June 4, 1997).

Henry, Sarah. "One on One: Should Doctors Help Patients Die? An Interview with Timothy Quill." 11 *Hippocrates* 26–28 (1997).

In Re Guardianship of Sharon Kowalski, Case No. C2-91-1047, 1991 Minn. App. LEXIS 1196 (unpublished opinion).

In Re Quinlan, 70 N.J. 10, 355 A.2d 647 (1976).

Kindelan, Kieron, and Gerry Kent. "Concordance Between Patients' Information Preferences and General Practitioners' Peceptions." 1 *Psychology and Health* 399–409 (1987).

Lee, Melinda A., Heidi D. Nelson, Virginia P. Tilden, et al. "Legalizing Assisted-Suicide—Views of Physicians in Oregon." 334 *New England Journal of Medicine* 310–15 (1995).

Lidz, Charles W., Alan Meisel, Marian Osterweis, et al. "Barriers to Informed Consent." 99 *Annals of Internal Medicine* 539-43 (Oct. 1983).

Mitchell, J.L. "Cross-Cultural Issues in the Disclosure of Cancer." 6 *Cancer Practitioner* 153–60 (May/June 1998).

Morrison, R. Sean, Elizabeth W. Morrison, and Denise F. Glickman. "Physician Reluctance to Discuss Advance Directives: An Empiric Investigation of Potential Barriers." 154 *Archives of Internal Medicine* 2311 (Oct. 24, 1994).

Nilchaikovit, Tana, James M. Hill, and Jimmie C. Holland. "The Effects of Culture on Illness Behavior and Medical Care." 15 *General Hospital Psychiatry* 41–50 (1993).

Novack, Dennis H., Robin Plumer, Raymond L. Smith, et al. "Changes in Physicians' Attitudes Toward Telling the Cancer Patient." 241 *Journal of the American Medical Association* 897–900 (1979).

Ohnuki-Tierney, Emiko. *Illness and Culture in Contemporary Japan: An Anthropological View.* Cambridge, MA: Cambridge University Press, 1984.

Oken, Donald. "What to Tell Cancer Patients." 175 *Journal of the American Medical Association* 1120–28 (1961).

Procanik v. Cillo, 97 N.J. 339, 478 A.2d 755 (1984).

Reich, Warren Thomas, editor-in-chief. *Encyclopedia of Bioethics,* 2nd ed., Vol 1. New York: Macmillan, 1995.

Robertson, J. A. *American Civil Liberties Union: Rights of the Critically Ill.* New York: Ballinger, 1983.

Roe v. Wade, 410 U.S. 113 (1973).

Sasako, M. "Getting Informed Consent in Clinical Trials on Japanese Cancer Patients." 23 *Gan To Kagaku Ryoho* 146–59 (Jan. 1996).

Schneiderman, Lawrence J., Richard Kronick, Robert M. Kaplan, et al. "Effects of Offering Advance Directives on Medical Treatments and Costs." 117 *Annals of Internal Medicine* 599–606 (Oct. 1, 1992).

Schoene-Seifert, Bettina, and James F. Childress. "How Much Should the Cancer Patient Know and Decide." 36 *CA-A Cancer Journal for Clinicians* 85 (March/April 1986).

Steinbrook, Robert, Bernard Lo, Jeffrey Moulton, et al. "Preferences of Homosexual Men with AIDS for Life-Sustaining Treatment." 314 *New England Journal of Medicine* 457–60 (1986).

Sterngold, James. "Japan's Health Care: Cradle, Grave and No Frills." *N.Y. Times*, Dec. 28, 1992, Sec. A, p. 1.

Stevens, C.A., and R. Hassan. "Management of Death, Dying and Euthanasia: Attitudes and Practices of Medical Practitioners in South Australia." 20 *Australian Journal of Medical Ethics* 41–46 (1994).

Superintendent of Belchertown v. Saikewicz, 373 Mass. 728, 370 N.E.2d 417 (Mass. 1977).

Thomsen, Ole O., Henrik R. Wulff, Alessandro Martin, et al. "What Gastroenterologists in Europe Tell Cancer Patients." 341 *Lancet* 473–76 (1993).

Turpin v. Sortini, 31 Cal. 3d 22, 643 P.2d 954 (1982).

van der Maas, Paul J., J.J.M. van Delden, L. Pijnenborg, et al. "Euthanasia and Other Medical Decisions Concerning the End of Life." 338 *Lancet* 669–74 (1991).

van der Maas, Paul J., Gerrit van der Wal, Ilinka Haverkate, et al. "Special Reports from the Netherlands: Euthanasia, Physician-Assisted Suicide, and Other Medical Practices Involving the End of Life in the Netherlands, 1990–1995." 335 *New England Journal of Medicine* 1699–705 (1996).

Ward, B.J., and P.A. Tate. "Attitudes among NHS Doctors to Requests for Euthanasia." 308 *British Medical Journal* 1332–34 (May 21, 1994).

Washington v. Glucksberg, 117 S.Ct. 2258 (1997).

Wilkes, Eric. "The Quality of Life." In *Palliative Care: The Management of Far Advanced Illness*. D. Doyle, ed. London & Philadelphia: Croom Helm & The Charles Press, 1984, pp. 9–19.

8

The Doctor's Role as Advocate

INTRODUCTION

> Not every patient can be saved, but his illness may be eased by the way the doctor responds to him—and in responding to him the doctor may save himself. But first he must become a student again; . . . he must see that his silence and neutrality are unnatural. It may be necessary to give up some of his authority in exchange for his humanity, but as the old family doctors knew, this is not a bad bargain.
>
> Anatole Broyard,
> *Intoxicated by My Illness*, p. 57

Doctors with compassion for their patients may need to become advocates for them. As Anatole Broyard suggests, this may require them to end their silence and, in doing so, to speak more carefully to and on behalf of their patients. Speaking up may require doctors to become political: as David Felton notes, "Politics is so heavily imbedded in all of medicine and research that it can't be extracted" (Moyers, 1993, p. 234). As discussed later, the increased regulation of health care professionals, including doctors who work for managed care organizations (MCOs), may bring doctors into the political arena. Doctors have already formed alliances with patients to fight the perceived abuses of MCOs.

Physicians may need to intervene to protect the best interests of their patients, not only in the hospital but in the community. For example, doctors should ensure that patients receive needed community-based services; this will require that doctors have the appropriate support from case managers and hospital social workers.

Advocacy might enable patients to remain productive so that they can continue to contribute to the world. But before patients can do this, doctors may need to counsel them regarding the best ways to "make the most" of their limitations and to cope with the circumstances created by their illnesses. Without "health," the ability to make such contributions is doubtful (even though some people's most significant contributions occur when they are ill). Advocacy should begin in the doctor's own practice and may extend to the world of politics—where the doctor may attempt to influence public policy so as to benefit patients.

The model for advocacy proposed here is based on a heightened respect for the value of patients. It shows patients that doctors really care about them.

ADVOCACY AS A MEANS TO PROVIDE BETTER SERVICES

Advocacy within the Doctor's Practice

Doctors can start advocating for patients by looking at how they treat those in their practices. They should consider whether

- they respect their patients' right to make health-related decisions.
- their decisions are patient-centered.
- they should know more about their patients and their families.
- they need to improve their ability to relate to patients and more effectively counsel them.

Deferring to the right of patients to make health-related decisions may be difficult for doctors with high power needs:[1] Such doctors may prefer to exert their power over patients and tell them what medications to take or what procedures to undergo. Many patients will not appreciate this authoritative "style."

Medical staff must be sensitive to the fact that their work should be patient-centered and based on the needs of patients, not the convenience of the staff. Patient-centered staff make matters easier for patients: helping them to overcome their limitations, enlisting the support of others to help patients (e.g., helping patients find support groups), or working with families—so that they understand the nature of the disease and its progression.

Getting to Know Patients and Their Families

Consider some of the practical benefits of doctors' getting to know more about their patients and their families:

- One physician treated several women for pelvic and abdominal pain, all of whom had attempted suicide. As this doctor got to know her patients better, they confided that they had all been sexually abused (Janiger & Goldberg, 1993, p. 48).
- One practitioner is noted for his "informal relations" with patients. He says, "My goal is to really know my patients, know how they think, know the way they are, know their character, so that when they're out of character I know it. . . . I want to know, does their life work?" (ibid., p. 55).

The preceding anecdotes illustrate that when doctors know their patients better, they often learn facts that will let them meet their patients' medical needs more efficiently.

Counseling Patients

[I]n the art . . . of medicine, a sociologically inescapable facet of treatment—often irrespective of how much is clinically known or unknown—is frequently that of somehow getting the patient and his family to accept, "put up with," or "make the best of" the socially and physically disadvantageous consequences of illness.

Fred Davis,
"Uncertainty in Medical Prognosis, Clinical and Functional,"
in *Medical Men and Their Work*, p. 244

In counseling patients, doctors can also provide them with hope. They should be mindful of Frankl's advice: "No man can ever know what life still holds in store for him, or what magnificent hour may still await him" (Frankl, 1955, p. 61). Chronic and terminally ill patients may feel that their lives are not meaningful because they can no longer do what they once did. Doctors can help patients realize that illness does not mean that their lives no longer have any value or significance and that no further interesting and important experiences await them. If nothing else, the challenge of coping with illness can be a significant accomplishment in itself.

Some patients may be understandably despondent when considering what they have done with their lives. They may have indeed "wasted" time when they were healthy. Doctors can remind such patients that the future still awaits them. They can still become great. According to Frankl, "The greatness of a life can be measured by the greatness of a moment: the height of a mountain range is not given by the height of some valley, but by that of the tallest peak" (ibid., p. 49).

Advocacy within the Hospital Setting

Doctors can play a valuable role ensuring that hospital staff (including nursing staff, respiratory and physical therapists, social workers) remain sensitive to patients' needs. As Emry Gorski's interview at the end of this chapter indicates, hospital staff can be a great source of frustration to patients when they are incompetent, insensitive, or inflexible. They may blindly apply hospital rules and not tailor them to individual situations that may sometimes require more flexible application.

Because the patient's physician is ultimately responsible for the patient's care in the hospital, the doctor must ensure that all hospital staff carry out their duties competently and compassionately. This is a tall order to fill. But proper patient care demands it.

Staff Insensitivity to Patients

Much of a hospital staff's insensitivity to patients may result from misunderstanding the patient's experience and the patient's needs and expectations. Rather than reacting angrily toward an angry patient, staff need to understand the source of the anger and then empathize with the patient— viewing the situation from the patient's perspective. Persons with AIDS may have anger to vent for some of these reasons:

- They may have been disowned by their families because they are homosexual and/or have AIDS.
- They may have recently been fired from their jobs or evicted from their apartments or have litigated insurance coverage disputes.
- They may not yet accept their diagnosis and still resent having such a debilitating condition at a young age.

Advocacy within the Community

If we really believe the patient is the center of the healing process, then we have to go after whatever circumstances contribute to a bad outcome. And if that means taking social action, fine, then let's take social action to change some of those factors that have an adverse impact on a patient's ability to recover from disease.

David Felten
quoted in Moyers,
Healing and the Mind, pp. 233–34

Doctors may especially need to advocate for patients on public aid and for those who are homeless, mentally ill, or suffering from diseases with social stigma (e.g., AIDS). This advocacy role will often take the form of getting services for clients. It may require that doctors offer testimony and attend meetings with legislators about bills that may affect these and other populations of patients.

In order for patients to get appropriate services in their communities, doctors may need to advocate for and assist them in obtaining housing, psychiatric services, or medications.

Assisting Patients to Obtain Housing. Many poor patients are discharged from hospitals (including psychiatric hospitals) without appropriate housing or care. It is inhumane to discharge those with serious illnesses to unstable housing situations or shelters—such individuals may be put out into the cold during winter months, for example.

Assisting Patients to Obtain Psychiatric Services. Psychiatric services have become virtually impossible to obtain: in most states, the mentally ill are turned down when they voluntarily seek psychiatric services at hospitals and community mental health centers (see the interview with Lucille Doty, a 63-year-old woman who remains active in her community despite her diagnosis with schizophrenia at the age of 22, at the end of the chapter). Furthermore, it is difficult for the mentally ill to be involuntarily admitted to psychiatric hospitals unless they meet overly restrictive legal criteria—that they are likely to harm themselves or others.

Assisting Patients to Obtain Medications. Many patients face the choice of paying for food or for medications. The inability to afford medications will cause many to discontinue their use (Lurie, Ward, Shapiro, et al., 1986). This situation has recently become a problem for people with AIDS (Pear, 1997). Physicians could work to ensure that state AIDS drug assistance programs continue to pay for protease inhibitors, that class of drugs which reduces the amount of HIV in a patient's body and are considered to have decreased the mortality rate of people with HIV. Some states have refused to pay for any of the protease inhibitors, and others have restricted the number of protease inhibitors they will pay for (see Kolata, 1996).[2]

CHALLENGING THE "CORPORATE MODEL" OF HEALTH CARE SET BY MANAGED CARE

Ensuring that patients have access to appropriate health care has increasingly become a challenge in light of current corporate models of health care such as MCOs—and including health maintenance organizations (HMOs).[3]

Managed care is often perceived as the corporate solution to controlling the escalating costs of health care. Although some economists have argued that an HMO's costs (including premiums charged to patients) could be controlled by the increased competition for business, others who have studied HMOs in several market economies have explained why HMOs do not control their costs (Hsiao, 1994); a major reason they do not is that "consumers do not necessarily have time, information or the presence of mind to engage in price shopping when faced with an emergency or striking illness" (ibid.). As a result, health care consumers do not seek out the most competent and cost-efficient doctor or group practice. Furthermore, even if HMOs were able to contain their costs, they would do so by selecting low-risk customers who have the ability to pay. Such practices that overtly discriminate against indigent "high-risk" consumers of health care do not lower overall health care expenditures—they merely shift the cost of caring for the sickest patients to the local, state, and federal governments.

For-profit HMOs are designed to be as profitable as possible. Unfortunately, a large percentage of the profits of such corporations go to executives—chief executive officers of HMOs earn an average 62 percent more than CEOs of other corporations of similar size (Bodenheimer, 1996)—rather than being reinvested for better services for patients. By the 1990s a small number of large nonprofit HMOs (e.g., Harvard Community Health Plan, Group Health Cooperative of Puget Sound) continued to spend 90 percent or more on direct patient care (Anders, 1996, p. 62). In contrast, by 1994 the largest publicly traded HMOs spent 76.6 percent of their premiums on direct patient care (ibid.). Advertising and marketing tactics of HMOs are also designed to ensure their profitability—and a steady stream of healthy patients. The highlight box, "HMO

Abuses in Marketing and Advertising," illustrates some questionable tactics that have been used by some HMOs.

How Managed Care Jeopardizes the Physician/Patient Relationship

As many medical practitioners become preoccupied with the profitability of their practices (particularly those who work for MCOs), the rights of patients are being adversely affected. The following factors can seriously compromise the best interest of patients:

- Gag clauses in HMO contracts that prohibit doctors from disclosing to patients services and treatments not provided by the HMO: As discussed later, such clauses also encourage doctors not to make referrals in order to contain costs for specialists ("H.M.O. Gag Rules," 1996).
- The pressure to reduce the time spent as an inpatient in a hospital is tremendous and growing (see the interview with Emry Gorski at the end of the chapter). In response to public demands, some states have felt it necessary to pass laws to prevent women who have just delivered children from being discharged too quickly from hospitals. The Breast Cancer Patient Protection Act of 1997, which would require insurance companies to provide at least 48 hours of inpatient hospital care after a mastectomy and a minimum of 24 hours after lymph node dissection for breast cancer treatment, is currently pending in the United States House of Representatives and Senate.
- Efforts by employers to become self-insured so that they can specifically cap payment for HIV-related conditions:[4] Self-insured employers have also typically capped payment for health-related expenses associated with chemical dependency and mental illness (see Vogel, 1987).

Although managed care may be perceived to have an "up" side (e.g., cost control measures and the ability to ensure that timely preventive care is offered) (Anders, 1996, p. 13), it has many "down" sides (discussed later).

MCOs are postured to make significant advances in preventive care despite several known barriers in implementing such care (Thompson, 1996). For example, prominent barriers to prevention include the facts that

- the current health system views physicians' duties as responding to symptoms (whereas in preventive care the goal is to promote the health of asymptomatic individuals) (ibid.).
- time constraints cause physicians to respond rather than to initiate (ibid.).

The amount of information HMOs collect should enable them to assess the effectiveness of their programming. Consider some of the following cost-effective programs introduced by MCOs that are also excellent health policy models:

- United Healthcare of Milwaukee, Wisconsin, invested $80,000 in a drug-education program for Medicaid mothers-to-be and found it reduced neonatal intensive-care admissions—an expense of $200,000 per case—by 50 percent (Grandjean, 1997).

- Group Health Cooperative of Puget Sound (GHC)—a member-owned HMO[5]—under a five-year-old program provides frequent blood tests, foot exams, and eye exams to its 10,000 diabetic subscribers. In 1997, the number of diabetics who underwent amputation dropped from 4 per 1,000 members to 2.7 per 1,000 members (Spragins, 1998). GHC has also conducted prevention campaigns, among others, to reduce tobacco use among its enrollees and to persuade enrollees to use helmets (Thompson, 1996). GHC reports a smoking cessation rate (defined as complete abstinence for at least one month, one year after the program) between 29 and 31 percent depending on whether smokers are counseled individually over the phone or in group sessions (ibid.). And it attributes the 67 percent decrease in head injury rates to its campaign to persuade enrollees to wear helmets (ibid.).

However, the medical literature also contains some discussion of HMOs' failed preventive efforts (Burack, Gimotty, George, et al., 1998; Simon, Gimotty, Coombs, et al., 1998; Thrall, McCloskey, Spivak, et al., 1998). For example, an HMO serving predominantly inner-city African American women sent enrollees a letter encouraging them to have a mammogram; yet only 48 percent of the women who received this letter actually had a mammogram (Simon, Gimotty, Coombs, et al., 1998). Another HMO, which sent women a letter to remind them to obtain a Pap smear, concluded that the letter had a "limited impact" on persuading patients to visit their HMO or to get a Pap smear (Burack, Gimotty, George, et al., 1998). Furthermore, only a very small percentage of female adolescents enrolled in Massachusetts HMOs received either a Pap smear or testing for a sexually transmitted disease despite professional guidelines recommending these tests (Thrall, McCloskey, Spivak, et al., 1998).

Although some HMOs have been engaged in constructive endeavors, such as the prevention efforts mentioned, many for-profit HMOs have come under increasing criticism for a variety of policies that threaten the patient/physician relationship. The following section summarizes major HMO policies that have come under the public's scrutiny.

How HMOs Regulate the Contractual Obligations of Physicians

HMOs hire groups of doctors whom they expect to comply with many contractual obligations—including those that provide doctors with "financial incentives" to undertreat certain conditions. These incentives are designed to ensure that the HMO remains highly profitable. The following are typical examples of these financial incentives:

- A bonus arrangement for doctors—the amount of the bonus depends on the profits doctors earn from their patient base: Some HMOs however, forbid their doctors to disclose to patients bonuses that they are paid for holding down costly referrals to specialists ("H.M.O. Gag Rules," 1996).
- A "sliding scale" salary for doctors, including pay cuts if their HMO is not profitable (Pear, 1996c).
- A rule that muzzles doctor/patient conversations about proper treatment practices ("H.M.O. Gag Rules," 1996).

- A standard of care, preestablished by the HMO, often expressly prepared to limit care.

Not only will those financial incentives deter doctors from advocating for their patients' needs, but some additional clauses in a doctor's contract with an HMO will foreclose any patient-related advocacy. For example, the following language is typical of some contracts:

Physician shall take no action nor make any communication that undermines or could undermine the confidence of enrollees, potential enrollees, their employers, plan sponsors or in the quality of care [the HMO's] enrollees receive. (Pear, 1996a)

A startling consequence of such contractual language is that physicians have been fired from MCOs for advocating for procedures or consultations that they consider medically necessary (see "Managed Scare," 1994/95).

HMO ABUSES IN MARKETING AND ADVERTISING

In advertising and marketing their services to enroll patients, HMOs have often used illegal practices. For example, HMOs already illegally ask 43 percent of Medicare applicants about their health status (Woolhandler & Himmelstein, 1995).

There are many "legal" ways in which HMOs can screen-out costly patients; for example, health plans can avoid "high-risk" enrollees by not contracting with providers known for specializing in certain high-risk conditions (Luft, 1996) or by engaging in practices referred to as *cream skimming* or *cherry picking* (Bodenheimer & Grumbach, 1996)—enrolling only healthy patients by, for instance, enrolling the elderly who regularly attend aerobics classes.

In order to induce patients to join their HMO during an enrollment period, some have signed up many local doctors, then, after patients have joined the network, HMOs pare down their list of physicians (Cropper, 1996). Furthermore, the listing of doctors or hospitals in an HMOs network does not always mean that patients enrolled in the HMO can choose that doctor or hospital (ibid.). For example, self-insured employers often offer what is called a "limited provider network," which buys access to some, not all, of the HMOs doctors (ibid.).

How Managed Care Jeopardizes Quality of Care

There are many practices of HMOs that will ultimately decrease the quality of care at least for sick individuals, including those who are terminally ill or have chronic conditions. These practices include using smaller portions of patient premiums for health-related services, while larger portions of the premiums are reserved for stockholders and the salaries of HMO managers and chief executive officers;[6] refusing to pay for what many would consider bona fide emergency treatment; designing standards of care that actually limit care; eliminating certain appeal rights designed to ensure quality of care; and limiting access to specialists.

Refusing to Pay for Bona Fide Emergency Treatment. HMOs refuse to pay for between 10 and 30 percent of all emergency room visits (Anders, 1996, p. 134). Consequently, they leave members liable for the charges, alleging that there was no legitimate emergency. HMOs have come under tremendous public pressure to change such practices.

Activists have challenged the ways in which HMOs determine whether a situation is an emergency or nonemergency. They have noted that patients vary in how they may report symptoms: some patients may be confused or panicky; others may be stoic; some may not explain their symptoms clearly; and others may not fit neatly into a particular emergency category (ibid., p. 141). Some HMOs have not even encouraged members to call 911 in an emergency. In a survey of Chicago HMOs, only 3 of 25 plans informed members it was permissible to dial 911 in an emergency (ibid., p. 148). Legislation in several states has often defined an emergency—a situation a reasonable person would consider serious or life-threatening—so as to bolster patients' claims that their visits to emergency rooms were appropriate.

Developing Standards of Care Designed to Limit Care. HMOs often have developed standards of care that, in some cases, are designed to limit care. Alternatively, standards of care may be indirectly affected when HMOs "shop around" for services at the cheapest price; as a result, patients enrolled in HMOs cannot select doctors or hospitals of their choice even when they have particular expertise.[7] Consequently, it may be no surprise that patients undergoing heart surgery were less likely to die if they had commercial insurance versus HMO coverage (ibid., p. 107). Patients' quality of care may also be jeopardized when they lose certain rights to appeal an HMOs decision. Medicare beneficiaries who enroll in HMOs lose important appeal rights only available under traditional Medicare (Schodolski, 1994)—even though the HMO may have its own internal system for appeals.

Limiting Access to Specialists. When patients require specialized care and/or consultations with specialists are critical to diagnose and treat patients, the "gatekeeper theory" of managed care is sometimes a significant threat to care. A *gatekeeper*—usually but not always a physician—performs an initial screening or assessment of the patient's situation. In companies that provide mental health services, the gatekeeper is the case manager. This individual, often a nurse or social worker, has authority to determine the type of professional who is seen (e.g., psychiatrist, psychologist, social worker, or counselor) as well as the extent of the treatment (Anders, 1996, pp. 156–57). Gatekeepers determine whether patients will even be referred to another physician and, if so, the type of physician they will see. They are used to prevent overtreatment and to limit referral to specialists.

How Managed Care Compromises Patient Confidentiality

Because confidentiality has often been the cornerstone of the physician/patient relationship, especially in the context of psychotherapy, any threat to this relationship is of concern to many patients. The managed care establishment threatens patient confidentiality (Corcoran & Winslade, 1994; Lewin, 1996); in order to keep down their costs, for example, MCOs have sought to review the files—or to have utilization review companies review the files—of patients to assess the appropriateness of the treatment provided for the particular problem, the nature of the patient's progress, and the necessity of continued treatment (Corcoran & Winslade, 1994).

MCOs allege that they have a legitimate interest in assuring that the services they purchase are necessary, reasonably priced, and not fraudulent (ibid., p. 360). As a result, some have proposed the following innovations to resolve the obvious fact that utilization review jeopardizes the patient's confidentiality (particularly in the mental health context, where the communication between psychotherapists and patients has been given special protection):

- MCOs should be included among those groups obliged to protect the patient's confidentiality: Access to the patient's medical information would be permissible only if there were an assurance that it would be kept confidential. Obviously, MCOs would be required to develop methods to protect the patient's identity (at least for patients receiving mental health services) as well as the patient's information.
- Patients should be allowed to participate in the utilization review process by providing information to those conducting the utilization review. This would allow them to control any information known about them (ibid., p. 362).
- To the extent that patients may not participate in the utilization review process, they should be counseled to permit disclosure of as little information as needed for a decision to be reached (ibid.). This is important since forms providing for the general release of information often do not inform patients of the third parties to whom the information might be disclosed (ibid., p. 358).
- Standards should be adopted for the amount of information insurers or utilization reviewers need, who will have access to it, how it will be kept secure, and how long it will be retained (Sabin, 1997).

Solutions for the Reform of Our Health Care System and of Managed Care

Some have suggested that rising per capita expenditures for health care in the United States would best be controlled by a single-payer system capable of eliminating spending for "administrative expenses," which represent an estimated 20 percent of health care costs. See the discussion in the highlight box for consideration of the Canadian health care system, a model of a single-payer system.

The managed care industry is currently regulated in some fashion. The Health Care Financing Administration (HCFA), a division of the United States Department of Health and Human Services, regulates Medicare HMOs—with over five million enrollees (see Colenda, Banazak, & Mickus, 1998; Pear, 1996c; Sage, 1996). HCFA policies and regulations affecting Medicare HMOs have included the following:

- Beginning January 1, 1997, HCFA promulgated rules to "protect patients against improper clinical decisions made under the influence of strong financial incentives" (Pear, 1996c). For example, the rules required HMOs to disclose their financial incentive arrangements to Medicare beneficiaries who requested them. They also required doctors (not HMOs) to carry insurance that would limit the amount of money lost on any particular patient (ibid.). The rules specified that a doctor group receiving fixed monthly payments to care for 7,000 patients must have insurance to cover most of the cost of "referral services" above $40,000 for any patient (ibid.). This rule should be useful in ensuring that doctors whose salaries are tied to the need to limit patient services—because the cost of referral is deducted from the doctor's salary—will not base patient-related decisions on the physician's financial interest.
- Medicare HMO patients with dementia must receive certain psychiatric services (Colenda, Banazak, & Mickus, 1998).

HCFA policies and regulations are believed to influence standards set for the entire managed care industry (Pear, 1996b) and, to that extent, seem to have significant potential for reform.

The managed care industry can also be reformed via the legislative process. Legislative efforts to reform MCOs have been under way for several years. Since early 1997, about 27 states have adopted patient-protection laws (Spragins, 1998). Through September 1996, 16 states passed legislation that prohibited "gag" clauses in health plans ("Ban All H.M.O.'s from Muzzling Doctors," 1996). California has even attempted to put some brakes on investor driven health care; in Medi-Cal managed care contracts, the state has limited the administrative expenses and the profit margin of HMOs (Sage, 1996 *citing* California's W&I Code, § 14464 [1995]). Over the next decade, legislation to regulate managed care will be needed in several of the following critical areas:

- Because it is not currently cost-effective for MCOs to provide high-quality care to the elderly, protective legislation will be necessary in order to protect this vulnerable class.
- Experts agree that Medicare HMOs have little incentive to provide high-quality care to the sickest elderly because "success only attracts more high-cost patients" (Spragins, 1998, p. 66).
- Because other sick and "specialized populations" with expensive medical conditions will require particular expertise to treat, they will also be vulnerable if treated by the MCO system. A Canadian study has found that 50 percent of men with AIDS (or who contracted AIDS while in the study) lived for 17 months under managed care versus men who sought medical care in a traditional fee-for-service arrangement who lived for 30 months, almost twice as long (Hosein, 1996). Many people with HIV/AIDS have already reported significant problems with HMOs, in particular, finding specialists competent to treat their conditions, restrictions on drugs available through the plan, and limitations on coverage of pharmaceuticals ("AIDS Advocates, Caregivers Must Play Major Role in Managed Care Debates," 1996). Some HMOs have also instituted *pharmacy risk sharing* in which physicians

are placed on a monthly drug budget—they are penalized if they exceed the budget and rewarded if they stay below it (Johannes, 1997). Because AIDS-related drugs may cost $1000 per month, pharmacy risk sharing will have an adverse impact on people with HIV/AIDS.

SAVING HEALTH CARE COSTS VIA A SINGLE-PAYER SYSTEM—THE CANADIAN HEALTH CARE SYSTEM

Some have argued that a single-payer health care system would be the most effective way to control the escalation of health care costs and to provide universal access to health insurance (Himmelstein, Woolhandler, & The Writing Committee of the Working Group on Program Design, 1989; McDermott, 1994; Schiff, Bindman, Brennan, et al., 1994). The health care system in Canada is an example of a single-payer system. Apparently, Canada achieves "high quality care for all" at a cost of 40–50 percent less than the United States (Schiff, 1994). And Canadian consumers are satisfied with their health system, according to a Harris poll—Canada was the highest among 10 nations surveyed (the United States was the lowest) (ibid.). More recently, 37 percent of Canadians have rated the quality of health care in Canada as good or excellent (Sibbald, 1998).

The Canadian system eliminates much administrative waste: administrative costs are held to 10 percent. In the United States, 20 percent of health care costs are for administrative expenses—including overhead expenses and costs "for determination of eligibility, for selling costs and commissions to insurance agents, for multiple and complex filling out of forms for reimbursement, for maintaining large and complicated billing systems, for carrying charges on accounts receivable, [and] for multiple bureaucracies both governmental and commercial" (Lee, 1982, p. 299; *see also* Angell, 1993).

In the Canadian system, any outlay for capital expenditures, such as for the construction of new hospitals, is controlled. Historically, the United States had no cost containment for capital expenditures—if a hospital wished to build a new wing, loan payments for the capital expenditure were added to the Blue Cross bill (Bodenheimer, 1990). This resulted in overexpansion of the hospital sector. Patients bore the costs of such overexpansion. For example, with the average hospital over 60 percent occupied, and with empty beds costing half as much to operate as full ones, the cost of empty hospital beds was added to the bill of hospital patients (ibid.).

Current Problems with the Canadian Health Care System

The Canadian health care system, however, is not currently without problems (DePalma, 1996; Sibbald, 1998). The cost of maintaining the system has apparently reduced the quality of care. Canadians who have been examined by their family doctor may expect to wait an average of 10 weeks to see a specialist (DePalma, 1996). And 50 percent of Canadian physician respondents cited a lack of well-equipped medical facilities as a problem (Blendon, Donelan, Leitman, et al., 1993). Doctors also believe they are being unfairly held responsible—or financially punished—for the government's decreasing commitment to funding national health care.

Doctors are "protesting" the perceived deficiencies of Canada's health care system. These protests have included strikes (not uncommon in other single-payer systems [Saltman, 1992]), legal action, and even legislative reform. Rural doctors, for example, are disgruntled over the typical 80-hour weeks they have been expected to work because of the serious maldistribution of physicians in some areas (Sibbald, 1998). As a result, many rural doctors have withdrawn their hospital services (ibid.). Essentially, they are on strike against the government.

The reason that the quality of care may be declining in Canada is related to the government's decreased financial commitment to running the system: the federal government, which used to finance 50 percent of the cost of maintaining the system, now contributes 32 percent—shifting a greater percentage of the financial burden to the provinces (ibid.).

To address the financial repercussions that they have been expected to assume, doctors have also brought legal action. The Manitoba Medical Association (MMA), representing the interests of 2,000 doctors, has sued Manitoba Health to recover $7 million in fees and $27 million in special damages, including damages for "broken promises" by the province of Manitoba (ibid.). The allegation for damages based on a "broken promise" is premised on what doctors have perceived as the government's bad faith negotiation; for four years the MMA worked with Manitoba Medical Services Council and a joint management team consisting of government officials and public and medical professionals, to generate cost-saving measures of $5 million to $6 million dollars per year (ibid.). A new health minister was appointed shortly after these negotiations, yet these cost-saving measures were never implemented (ibid.). But the province still wants doctors to absorb any cost overruns.

One disgruntled doctor is seeking more significant reform of Canada's single–payer system. Dr. Jack Chaoulli, a physician in Quebec, proposes that doctors be obliged to work a certain number of hours in the public health care system but have the option of working privately for another set period (ibid.). Such a system exists in France and Germany.

Cutbacks in Canada's public health system have imposed some financial impact on doctors. The Alberta Medical Association says that doctors' fees have fallen 30 percent behind inflation (ibid., p. 1508). But Canadian doctors' salaries have been lower than those of their United States counterparts for some time. According to a study conducted between 1971 and 1985, after adjusting for inflation, the fees of physicians in Canada decreased 18 percent as those of physicians in the United States rose 22 percent ("Canadian Health Insurance," 1991).

From 1992 to 1995, about 2,500 doctors left Canada, many for the United States (DePalma, 1996). Primary care physicians often move to the United States as a result of new and "aggressive" recruitment efforts (Wilson, Woodhead-Lyons, & Moores, 1998).

Patients using the legal system to address harm or injury they have suffered at the hands of MCOs may have limited remedies (Sage, 1996). This is because a federal law passed in 1974, the Employee Retirement Income Security Act (ERISA), exclusively regulates "welfare benefits" such as health coverage—as a result of this "exclusive regulation," ERISA plans are shielded from state laws that relate to employee benefits plans (ibid.). Therefore, ERISA negates many legal remedies that might arise under state law, such as claims for breach of a contract due to "bad faith" or claims for emotional distress (ibid., p. 12). Money damages available to a claimant filing a suit for violation of ERISA do not include punitive damages and are unlikely to include damages for "pain and suffering" (ibid.).

Lawyers representing patients, however, have begun to sue HMOs and to attack the traditional status quo of ERISA preemption. Consider some of the novel legal arguments that have been advanced (and have succeeded) and others that are likely to be advanced (and may succeed):

- Because MCOs often promise to render "comprehensive services for prepaid premiums," any bad health outcome might be viewed as a denial of "medically necessary" benefits or the result of medical malpractice. The first type of claim would be for breach of contract,[8] and the second claim for medical malpractice, would be a claim for a *tort*—a legally recognized "injury" for which money damages are appropriate (Prosser, Wade, & Schwartz, 1982).
- In situations in which doctors may not have the best interests of patients in mind because of a financial conflict of interest, some court decisions in other contexts suggest that physicians will be obliged to disclose their conflict of interest.[9]
- Not only does case law on the physician/patient relationship firmly establish a doctor's high level of care owed the patient,[10] the result of the fiduciary relationship between doctor and patient, but it is beginning to suggest that in the context of MCOs, third parties such as utilization review companies are also legally accountable for their actions.[11]

CHAPTER SUMMARY

Increasingly, patients expect their doctors to advocate for their many needs. This may require that doctors become political, lobbying for legislation sympathetic to patients' rights. Doctors and patients have lobbied successfully against various standards adopted by for-profit HMOs.

The HMO evolved during President Nixon's presidency "as a policy alternative to blunt the drive for national health insurance." HMOs are often considered to be able to deliver effective preventive health care services. Several HMOs have reported making inroads in reducing amputations in their patients with diabetes (by recommending regular foot care and monitoring blood sugar levels), reducing smoking among enrollees, and increasing helmet use and, thereby, reducing head injuries of members.

Historically, many HMOs were nonprofit; in the mid– to late 1980s, however, the for-profit HMO came to dominate the field and with it many policies that were adverse to the best interests of patients, including gag clauses in the contracts of doctors employed by HMOs; refusal to pay for bona fide emergency treatment; design of standards of care aimed to limit care; restriction of access to specialists; and compromising of patient confidentiality.

Gag clauses have both prohibited doctors from disclosing to patients services and treatments provided by the HMO and discouraged doctors from making referrals in order to hold down the cost of specialists. With regard to the latter provisions, many HMO contracts stipulate that doctors will receive bonuses if they limit care and, therefore, increase the HMOs profit margin.

Studies show that HMOs have refused to pay for 10–30 percent of enrollee visits to emergency rooms. As a result, legislation in several states has defined an emergency as a situation a reasonable person would consider serious or life-threatening. HMOs have also been accused of designing standards of care that actually limit appropriate care, and patient referrals to specialists have often been limited. HMOs have instituted gatekeepers to determine whether patients will be referred to another physician and, if so, to dictate the type of physician.

Reform of the MCO will occur at the legislative level and slowly, by court decisions that will uphold the rights of claimants injured by MCO practices. Even though the Employee Retirement Income Security Act bars legal remedies that might otherwise arise under state law—and limits money damages—courts have been willing to find HMOs liable under theories such as breach of contract. Some courts will likely take note of the conflict of interest of doctors who work for HMOs—obviously they may not act in their patients' best interests if they also have a financial incentive to withhold treatment.

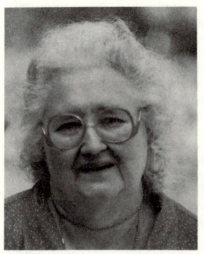

AN INTERVIEW WITH LUCILLE DOTY

I was diagnosed with schizophrenia in 1958 when I was 22 years old although at age 19 I knew I had problems because of academic difficulty in college. I also wandered around aimlessly with no real goals or plans for the future. With drug treatment (e.g., thorazine), I currently consider myself, and the control of my schizophrenia-associated symptoms, "almost average." I do not like to use the terms normal or abnormal.

Over a period of 40 years, I have been hospitalized in a mental hospital about 15 times. My longest admission was for 11 months. Two hospitalizations were for 6 months. Although I've had many psychiatrists, I've had long-term therapy with about three of them.

Psychotherapy has helped me throughout the years. Because my father was wealthy at the time I was diagnosed with schizophrenia, one of my first psychiatrists insisted that I have psychotherapy. One early treating psychiatrist helped me resolve the pain and problems from the past that were magnified in the present. In other words, by being able to resolve the psychological pain caused by past events, I was free to focus on the causes of my current pain. And years later another psychiatrist was able to motivate me to change my behavior for the better. For example, one time I spent my rent money and he made me sleepless for a night in order to impress upon me the need to use rent money only for rent.

I worked for 11 years as a secretary and bookseller. I was married for five years and have a daughter living in a state bordering the one in which I now live. I am also an insulin-dependent diabetic and each day I give myself an injection of insulin.

I was addicted to diet pills for 33 years until finally, with intervention of one psychiatrist, I ended this addiction. The psychiatrist who helped me with this notified state officials of my dependence on diet pills. These officials contacted all the doctors who prescribed me diet pills and, under threat of losing their licenses, they no longer prescribed these pills.

I take a rather high dose of thorazine for an outpatient. I do not believe I will be admitted to a psychiatric hospital again. I would, however, like to have psychotherapy. The last time I had psychotherapy was 12 years ago; it is practically impossible for me to get psychotherapy because of funding cuts for services for the mentally ill that started during the Reagan administration. The situation is more dreadful in states other than the one in which I live, however. Some states offer people "Greyhound therapy": they offer people who persistently seek services, like psychotherapy, a one-way bus ticket to any city in the United States.

I consider myself happy although I do not have much occasion for social contact in my current living situation. I live in a housing complex with other senior citizens who are mentally ill. Many are not too functional and for much of the day are like "zombies." I attend a local church regularly and have participated in many committees at the church. I am particularly interested in creative writing and wrote for a church newsletter, as well as writing and editing the newsletter compiled for members of my housing community. Additionally, I correspond with about 12 people on a regular basis.

My medical assistance is derived from public aid. While on public aid I've been hospitalized in both private and state-run mental hospitals. I've found the private hospitals to be quite good but the state-run hospitals to be quite bad, especially since many of the "lower echelon" staff seem to "run the hospital"— they treat the mentally ill as if they are naughty children and they gather them into "herds" to take them places. The nursing staff and psychiatrists spend little time with patients, the former because they are involved in charting patients' progress. Patients are removed, therefore, from people who are most likely to be sympathetic to their plight. Some psychiatrists in state-run mental hospitals do not seem to take much of an interest in the patients or in the place and they do not seem motivated to improve the situation. Years ago it seemed that mental health professionals working in mental hospitals tried to treat patients and improve their ability to function. The current situation seems quite different— hospitalizations are for shorter periods and the aim seems to be to just "stabilize" the patient, regardless of how functional the patient is.

I am the happiest now that I have ever been—and I started to be happier when I retired. I attribute this happiness to the medicine I now take, the therapy I have had, and the fact that I no longer work!

SUGGESTED READINGS

Isaac, Rael Jean, and Virginia C. Armat. *Madness in the Streets: How Psychiatry and the Law Abandoned the Mentally Ill.* New York: Free Press, 1990.

Torrey, E. Fuller. *Nowhere to Go: The Tragic Odyssey of the Homeless Mentally Ill.* New York: Harper & Row, 1988.

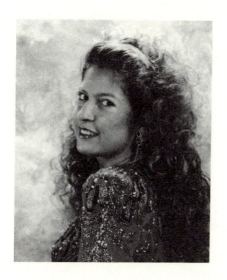

AN INTERVIEW WITH EMRY GORSKI

I am 35 years old and in 1980 I was diagnosed with allergic bronchopulmonary aspergilliosis (ABPA), a chronic fungal infection in my lungs. In 1988, I was diagnosed with several bacterial infections. Long-term steroid therapy to treat my ABPA has weakened my bones and I have suffered from both cracked ribs and a broken tail bone. ABPA is also associated with an inflamed pancreas (pancreatitis) and I frequently take the painkiller Demerol, to treat the pain associated with the pancreatitis.

I have had over 100 separate hospital admissions since being diagnosed with ABPA. When I am at home, the visiting nurse comes in twice a day to give me physical therapy so that fluid does not collect in my lungs.

I would characterize my relationship with my main treating physician, a pulmonary specialist, as "good"—my doctor understands my needs and concerns and I have trusted him. Very recently, however, my doctor has been under pressure from both my insurance company and the hospital to which he has admitted me to decrease the frequency and duration of my hospital admissions. This pressure, it seems, caused my doctor to yell at me and tell me to leave the hospital (at midnight!) during a recent admission. He then backtracked and said that I could remain through the night—feeling unwelcome, however, I signed myself out. My doctor apologized about a month after this incident.

I do not believe that insurance companies should be able to exert as much influence as they apparently do about the protocol for caring for patients. Of course, my insurance company does not want to cover the expenses associated with my care. I have offered to meet with the doctors for the insurance company to enable them to more effectively evaluate the need for my care. But needless to say they have not wanted to meet with me.

Although my relationship with my main treating physician is good, my relationship with many of the nursing staff and doctor-interns at the medical center where I obtain treatment is "strained" to "poor." I have gotten two nurses fired for medical errors they have made on my case.

Many of the hospital staff has been blatantly insensitive toward me. In my presence, one social worker commented that I sought hospitalization for "ridiculous" reasons and an intern intimated that I only sought hospitalization to obtain Demerol, to which I am addicted. Demerol seems to be the only medication that relieves the pain associated with my pancreatitis. Several of the nursing staff have implied that I should not leave my hospital room for fear that I am "contagious" and could infect other hospital patients. This insensitivity, which has obviously included much misunderstanding about the medical nature of my condition, will potentially be addressed through in-service training that my main treating physician has scheduled with the nursing staff. Because patients are treated by so many different staff members during any hospitalization, partly due to staff turnover, it has been difficult for my main treating physician to feel as though he can exert any "control" over staff sensitivity.

Even though my condition is quite serious and although I am quite sick, I often "look well." Unfortunately, one of the major myths about illness is that you have to look sick to be sick. I believe that based on this myth, many of the hospital personnel charged with my care believe that I may be a "malingerer" and that I am not as sick as I am.

I've had to live much of my life in the hospital. Over the years, I have become frustrated by the extent to which I've needed to "take charge" of my health care. I'm frustrated by many of the things I've had to say to correct situations that should be obvious to health-care professionals.

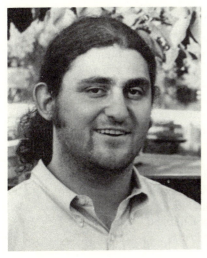

AN INTERVIEW WITH JEFF WINOGRAD

During the past 26 years, I have learned to deal with asthma which I have had my entire life. My asthma has always been average in severity. When a large attack occurs, I often require hospitalization. But I often spend months without much evidence of asthma, other than the daily use of an inhaler.

I have several constructive comments for the many pulmonary specialists who have treated me. First, I have the expectation that treatment for asthma should lead to my continued improvement and that I be less dependent on an inhaler to treat my shortness of breath. Second, I believe that doctors should listen more carefully to their patients, including to patients' expectations regarding treatment. Third, I am somewhat critical of what I have perceived as doctors' reluctance to explore non-drug-related treatments for control of asthma. Fourth, I would like to suggest a somewhat different role for the doctor, including the possibility of the doctor becoming the patient's friend.

Because I would like to be less dependent on an inhaler, I believe my doctor should continually help me to improve. I would ultimately like to be weaned off medication—either through an exercise program, breathing techniques, or even dietary changes.

I also believe that doctors should be more attentive to the patient's expectations regarding treatment. For example, I thought treatment would reduce the extent of my limitations. And my doctor's observation that there are professional sports figures with asthma who can play sports without any symptoms is not helpful, because I sometimes experience symptoms after climbing a flight of stairs. But when I describe such symptoms my doctors are befuddled because under the ideal conditions in which I am examined, I do not show any limited ability to breathe.

I do not believe that the various doctors who have treated me for asthma have been interested in non-drug-related treatments to control it. I have researched alternative means for controlling asthma. I found articles in the medical literature that reported cures with particular diets and was discouraged when my pulmonary specialists were not even aware of these articles.

Doctors should have a different role than the historic role they have had in the treatment of patients. I believe that doctors should be the friend and the coach of patients. When the doctor becomes the patient's friend, patients may be better able to control their asthma. Doctors' relationships with their patient must be organic and able to change and grow. A doctor should be open to hearing the specific needs of an individual that go beyond taking medication. Understanding patients' specific needs and how they would like to approach the treatment of their conditions will better assist doctors choose methods that will best suit patients. When doctors become the patient's coach, patients will be more motivated to comply with treatment regimens.

NOTES

1. Some believe that people with high power needs (including the need for status and recognition) become doctors.

2. Because of the cost of such drugs, states often reduce the number of drugs used to treat HIV/AIDS to the indigent (Pear, 1997). The AIDS Drug Assistance Programs (ADAPs) in four states do not cover any of the protease inhibitors (ibid.); in 10 states ADAPs have halted admissions, and seven others were rationing or no longer dispensing more expensive drugs (Silverstein, 1998, p. 68).

3. Paul Ellwood, who coined the term *HMO*, sold the concept to President Nixon "as a policy alternative to blunt the drive for national health insurance" (Himmelstein & Woodhandler, 1988, p. 498).

4. Although such practices are considered illegal under the Americans with Disabilities Act, this does not necessarily prevent employers from engaging in such practices.

5. GHC, which began in 1947, is the largest member-governed HMO in the country, with 483,000 members (Thompson, 1996). Its by-laws emphasize that special attention must be paid to preventive medicine (ibid.).

6. The wealthiest HMO tycoon is apparently Leonard Abramson, the founder of US Healthcare, whose estimated wealth is $1 billion (Anders, 1996, p. 58).

7. Consider the fact that the mortality rates vary widely among pediatric heart centers, from 3–4 percent to 25 percent (ibid., p. 107).

8. See *Dunn v. Praiss* (1985). In this case, the widow of a man who died of testicular cancer, which had spread to his liver, sued her deceased spouse's HMO, the HMO's physician charged with coordinating his care, and two physicians in a urologic group practice to which the patient was referred.

9. In *Moore v. Regents of the University of California* (1990), a case resolving a dispute of ownership of a cell line derived from the plaintiff's tissue, the Supreme Court of California stated, "A physician who is seeking a patient's consent for a medical procedure must, in order to satisfy his fiduciary duty and to obtain the patient's informed consent, disclose personal interests unrelated to the patient's health, whether research or economic, that may affect his medical judgment."

10. Although a doctor owes a patient a high level of "care," the reverse is not true because the patient is not legally considered to have any "special interest" in the welfare of the physician. Examples of cases that illustrate this high level of care doctors owe their patients include those in which HIV-positive doctors must disclose their HIV status to patients (*Behringer v. Princeton Medical Center*, 1991).

11. See *Wickline v. State of California*, 1986.

SUGGESTED READINGS

Anders, George. *Health Against Wealth: HMO's and the Breakdown of Medical Trust.* Boston: Houghton Mifflin, 1996.

Rodwin, Marc A. "Managed Care and Consumer Protection: What Are the Issues?" 26 *Seton Hall Law Review* 1007–54 (1996).

Sage, William M. "Health Law 2000: The Legal System and the Changing Health Care Market." 15 *Health Affairs* 9–27 (Fall 1996).

REFERENCES

"AIDS Advocates, Caregivers Must Play Major Role in Managed Care Debates" 11 *AIDS Alert* 49 (May 1996).

Anders, George. *Health Against Wealth: HMO's and the Breakdown of Medical Trust.* Boston: Houghton Mifflin, 1996.

Angell, Marcia. "How Much Will Health Care Reform Cost?" 328 *New England Journal of Medicine* 1778–79 (June 17, 1993).

"Ban All H.M.O.'s from Muzzling Doctors." *N.Y. Times*, Sept. 29, 1996, Sec. 4, p. 14.

Behringer v. Princeton Medical Center, 992 A.2d 1251, 249 N.J. Super 597 (N.J. Super. 1991).

Blendon, Robert J., Karen Donelan, Robert Leitman, et al. "Physicians' Perspectives on Caring for Patients in the United States, Canada, and West Germany." 328 *New England Journal of Medicine* 1011–16 (April 8, 1993).

Bodenheimer, Thomas. "The HMO Backlash—Righteous or Reactionary?" 335 *New England Journal of Medicine* 1601–4 (Nov. 21, 1996).

———. "Should We Abolish the Private Health Insurance Industry?" 20 *International Journal of Health Services* 199–220 (1990).

Bodenheimer, Thomas, and Kevin Grumbach. "Capitation or Decapitation: Keeping Your Head in Changing Times." 276 *Journal of the American Medical Association* 1025–31 (Oct. 2, 1996).

Broyard, Anatole. *Intoxicated by My Illness: And Other Writings on Life and Death.* New York: Fawcett Columbine, 1993.

Burack, Robert C., Phyllis A. Gimotty, Julie George, et al. "How Reminders Given to Patients and Physicians Affected Pap Smear Use in a Health Maintenance Organization: Results of a Randomized Controlled Trial." 82 *Cancer* 2391–400 (June 15, 1998).

California W&I Code § 14464 (1995).

"Canadian Health Insurance: Lessons for the United States." *Government Accounting Office Report* (June 1991).

Colenda, Christopher, Deborah Banazak, and Maureen Mickus. "Mental Health Services in Managed Care: Quality Questions Remain." 53 *Geriatrics* 49–52, 59–60, 63–64 (Aug. 1998).

Corcoran, Kevin, and William J. Winslade. "Eavesdropping on the 50-Minute Hour: Managed Mental Health Care and Confidentiality." 12 *Behavioral Sciences and the Law* 351–61 (1994).

Cropper, Carol Marie. "Spending It: The HMO Says the Doctor Is In. Is He Really?" *N.Y. Times*, Nov. 10, 1996, Sec. 3, p. 8.

Davis, Fred. "Uncertainty in Medical Prognosis, Clinical and Functional." In *Medical Men and Their Work.* E. Friedson and J. Lorber, eds. Chicago: Aldine Atherton, 1972, pp. 239–48.

DePalma, Anthony. "Doctor, What's the Pronosis? A Crisis for Canada." *N.Y. Times*, Dec. 15, 1996, Sec. 1, p. 3.

Dunn v. Praiss, 656 A.2d 413 (NJ 1985).

Frankl, Viktor E. *The Doctor and the Soul: An Introduction to Logotherapy.* New York: Alfred A. Knopf, 1955.

Grandjean, Patricia. "What You Need to Know about Managed Care." *Connecticut* 53–56, 79 (Feb. 1997).

Himmelstein, David U., and Steffie Woolhandler. "The Corporate Compromise: A Marxist View of Health Maintenance Organizations and Prospective Payment." 109 *Annals of Internal Medicine* 494–501 (Sept. 15, 1988).

Himmelstein, David U., Steffie Woolhandler, and The Writing Committee of the Working Group on Program Design. "A National Health Program for the United States: A Physician's Proposal." 320 *New England Journal of Medicine* 102–8 (Jan. 12, 1989).

"H.M.O. Gag Rules." *N.Y. Times*, Jan. 6, 1996, Sec. 1, p. 18 (editorial).

Hosein, Sein. "Testing: Survival Decreases under Managed Care." 8 *Treatment Update* (Canada) 72 (Oct. 1996).

Hsiao, William C. "'Marketization': The Illusory Magic Pill." 3 *Health Economics* 351–57 (1994).

Janiger, Oscar, and Philip Goldberg. *A Different Kind of Healing: Doctors Speak Candidly about Their Successes with Alternative Medicine.* New York: G. P. Putnam's Sons, 1993.

Johannes, Laura. "Some HMOs Now Put Doctors on a Budget for Prescription Drugs." *Wall Street Journal*, May 22, 1997, p. A1.

Kolata, Gina. "AIDS Patients Slipping Through Safety Net: Soaring Cost of Drugs Strains the Budgets of Programs and Patients." *N.Y. Times*, Sept. 15, 1996, Sec. 1, p. 24, col. 4.

Lee, Sidney S. "Health Policy, a Social Contract: A Comparison of the United States and Canada." 3 *Journal of Public Health Policy* 293–301 (Sept. 1982).

Lewin, Tamar. "A Loss of Confidence: A Special Report: Questions of Privacy Roil Arena of Psychotherapy." *N.Y. Times*, May 22, 1996, Sec. A, p. 1.

Luft, Harold S. "Modifying Managed Competition to Address Cost and Quality." 15 *Health Affairs* 23–38 (Spring 1996).

Lurie, Nicole, Nancy B. Ward, Martin F. Shapiro, et al. "Termination of Medi-Cal Benefits: A Follow-Up Study One Year Later." 314 *New England Journal of Medicine* 1266–68 (May 8, 1986).

"Managed Scare." *POZ*, Dec. 1994/Jan. 1995, p. 16 (letter to the editor).

McDermott, Jim. "Evaluating Health System Reform: The Case for a Single-Payer Approach." 271 *Journal of the American Medical Association* 782–84 (March 9, 1994).

Moore v. Regents of the University of California, 793 P.2d 479 (Cal. 1990), *cert. denied*, 499 U.S. 936 (1991).

Moyers, Bill. *Healing and the Mind.* New York: Doubleday, 1993.

Pear, Robert. "Expense Means Many Can't Get Drugs for AIDS." *N.Y. Times*, Feb. 16, 1997, p. 1, col. 5.

———. "Keeping Doctors Quiet." *N.Y. Times*, Sept. 22, 1996a, Sec. 4, p. 7.

———. "Laws Won't Let H.M.O.'s Tell Doctors What to Say." *N.Y. Times*, Sept. 17, 1996b, Sec. A, p. 12.

———. "U.S. Limits H.M.O.'s in Linking Bonuses to Cost Controls." *N.Y. Times*, Dec. 25, 1996c, Sec. A, p. 1.

Prosser, William L., John W. Wade, and Victor E. Schwartz. *Cases and Materials on Torts*, 7th ed. Mineola, NY: Foundation Press, 1982.

Sabin, James E. "What Confidentiality Standards Should We Advocate For in Mental Health Care, and How Should We Do It?" 48 *Psychiatric Services* 35–36, 41 (Jan. 1997).

Sage, William M. "Health Law 2000: The Legal System and the Changing Health Care Market." 15 *Health Affairs* 9–27 (Fall 1996).

Saltman, R.B. "Single-Source Financing Systems: A Solution for the United States?" 268 *Journal of the American Medical Association* 774–79 (Aug. 12, 1992).

Schiff, Gordon D. "Consumer Interest and Health Reform: The Logic of Withdrawal from Managed Competition." 28 *The Journal of Consumer Affairs* 234–54 (Winter 1994).

Schiff, Gordon D., Andrew B. Bindman, Troyen A. Brennan, et al. "A Better-Quality Alternative — Single–Payer National Health System Reform." 272 *Journal of the American Medical Association* 803–8 (Sept. 14, 1994).

Schodolski, Vincent J. "Tricky HMO Balance: Profits vs. Quality Care." *Chicago Tribune*, June 14, 1994, p. 1.

Sibbald, Barbara. "In Your Face: A New Wave of Militant Doctors Lashes Out." 158 *Canadian Medical Association Journal* 1505–9 (June 2, 1998).

Silverstein, Ken. "Sleeping with the Enemy: As Sky-High Drug Prices Bankrupt ADAPs, AIDS Advocates and Pharmaceutical Reps Make Strange Bedfellows." *POZ*, June 1998, pp. 66–69.

Simon, M.S., P.A. Gimotty, J. Coombs, et al. "Factors Affecting Participation in a Mammography Screening Program among Members of an Urban Detroit Health Maintenance Organization." 22 *Cancer Detection & Prevention* 30–38 (1998).

Spragins, Ellyn E. "Does Managed Care Work?" *Newsweek*, Sept. 28, 1998, pp. 61–63, 66.

Thompson, Robert S. "What Have HMOs Learned about Clinical Prevention Services? An Examination of the Experience of Group Health Cooperative of Puget Sound." 74 *Milbank Quarterly* 469–502 (1996).

Thrall, J.S., L. McCloskey, H. Spivak, et al. "Performance of Massachusetts HMOs in Providing Pap Smear and Sexually Transmitted Disease Screening to Adolescent Females." 22 *Journal of Adolescent Health* 184–89 (March 1998).

Vogel, Joan. "Containing Medical and Disability Costs by Cutting Unhealthy Employees: Does Section 510 of ERISA Provide a Remedy?" 62 *Notre Dame Law Review* 1024–62 (1987).

Wickline v. State of California, 192 Cal. App. 3d 1630 (Cal. Ct. App. 1986), *appeal dismissed*, 741 P.2d 613 (1987).

Wilson, Douglas R., Sandra C. Woodhead-Lyons, and David G. Moores. "Alberta's Rural Physician Action Plan: An Integrated Approach to Education, Recruitment and Retention." 158 *Canadian Medical Association Journal* 351–55 (Feb. 10, 1998).

Woolhandler, Steffie, and David U. Himmelstein. "Extreme Risk—The New Corporate Proposition for Physicians" (editorial). 333 *New England Journal of Medicine* 1706–8 (Dec. 21, 1995).

Index

About the Author

JAMES MONROE SMITH is a lawyer and scientist who has taught courses on the sociopolitical aspects of AIDS. He is the author of *AIDS and Society* (1996). He founded the AIDS Legal Council of Chicago, a nonprofit organization providing legal services and advocacy for persons affected by HIV/AIDS and, from 1988–1992, was its first executive director.